Atlas of Breast Pathology

To the memory of Iris Hamlin

Current Histopathology

Consultant Editor
Professor G. Austin Gresham, TD, ScD, MD, FRC Path.
Professor of Morbid Anatomy and Histology, University of Cambridge

Volume Seven

ATLAS OF
BREAST PATHOLOGY

BY ROSEMARY R. MILLIS

Consultant Histopathologist
Guy's Hospital and Imperial Cancer Research Fund Breast Cancer Unit
at Guy's and New Cross Hospitals
London

WKAP ARCHIEF

 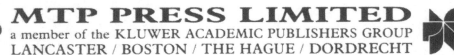
MTP PRESS LIMITED
a member of the KLUWER ACADEMIC PUBLISHERS GROUP
LANCASTER / BOSTON / THE HAGUE / DORDRECHT

Published by
MTP Press Limited
Falcon House
Queen Square
Lancaster, England

British Library Cataloguing in Publication Data

Millis, Rosemary R.
  Atlas of breast pathology.—(Current
histopathology; v. 7)
  1. Breast—Cancer—Diagnosis
  I. Title   II. Series
  616.99'44907   RC280.B8
  ISBN-13: 978-94-009-6591-1   e-ISBN-13: 978-94-009-6589-8
  DOI: 10.1007/978-94-009-6589-8

Library of Congress Cataloging in Publication Data

Millis, Rosemary R.
  Atlas of breast pathology.

  (Current histopathology; v. 7)
  Bibliography: p.
  Includes index.
    1.   Breast—Diseases—Diagnosis.   2.   Breast—
Cancer—Diagnosis.   3.   Histology, Pathological.
I.   Title. II.   Series.
[DNLM: 1. Breast diseases—
Pathology—   Atlases. W1 CU788JBA v. 7 / WP 17
M654a]   0
RG493.M55 1983   618.1'9075' 222   83–249ı
ISBN-13: 978-94-009-6591-1

Phototypesetting by Georgia Origination, Liverpool.
Colour origination by Replica Photo-Litho
Reproducers Limited, Stockport.
Printed by Cradley Print PLC, Warley, W. Midlands.
Bound by John Sherratt and Son Limited,
Manchester.

Contents

Current Histopathology Series

Consultant Editor's Note

At the present time books on morbid anatomy and histology can be divided into two broad groups: extensive textbooks often written primarily for students and monographs on research topics.

This takes no account of the fact that the vast majority of pathologists are involved in an essentially practical field of general Diagnostic Pathology providing an important service to their clinical colleagues. Many of these pathologists are expected to cover a broad range of disciplines and even those who remain solely within the field of histopathology usually have single and sole responsibility within the hospital for all this work. They may often have no chance for direct discussion on problem cases with colleagues in the same department. In the field of histopathology, no less than in other medical fields, there have been extensive and recent advances, not only in new histochemical techniques but also in the type of specimen provided by new surgical procedures.

There is a great need for the provision of appropriate information for this group. This need has been defined in the following terms.

(1) It should be aimed at the general clinical pathologist or histopathologist with existing practical training, but should also have value for the trainee pathologist.

(2) It should concentrate on the practical aspects of histopathology taking account of the new techniques which should be within the compass of the worker in a unit with reasonable facilities.

(3) New types of material, e.g. those derived from endoscopic biopsy should be covered fully.

(4) There should be an adequate number of illustrations on each subject to demonstrate the variation in appearance that is encountered.

(5) Colour illustrations should be used whereever they aid recognition.

The present concept stemmed from this definition but it was immediately realized that these aims could only be achieved within the compass of a series, of which this volume is one. Since histopathology is, by its very nature, systemized, the individual volumes deal with one system or where this appears more appropriate with a single organ.

Pathological conditions in the breast are common in the work of the diagnostic histopathologist. This atlas provides a comprehensive, modern view of the subject, with expert advice on the difficult problems in the distinction of neoplastic and non-neoplastic conditions. Students of pathology will find it a helpful concise atlas and it is a welcome addition to bench manuals for the histopathologist.

G. Austin Gresham
Cambridge

ERRATUM

Atlas of Breast Pathology

Page 87, under 'Secretory or Juvenile Carcinoma':
For 'Figures 15.9 and 15.10' read 'Figures 15.9–15.11'.

Page 87, under 'Lipid-rich Carcinoma':
For Figures 15.11 and 15.12' read 'Figure 15.12'.

Page 89: correct legend for Figure 15.11:
Figure 15.11 Secretory (juvenile) carcinoma. Another picture of the same tumour as that illustrated in Figures 15.9 and 15.10. In this field the very abundant eosinophilic material is predominantly extracellular. H & E × 240

Page 89: correct legend for Figure 15.12:
Figure 15.12 Lipid-rich carcinoma of the breast. A mammary carcinoma composed of closely-packed spheroidal cells with hyperchromatic nuclei and abundant, vacuolated, foamy cytoplasm. Frozen sections of unembedded tumour tissue stained with Oil Red O showed abundant lipid in almost all the cells. H & H × 240

Page 127, column 2: please delete the top three lines.

Introduction

The aim of this atlas is to illustrate the wide range of histological appearances which can be seen in breast biopsies and mastectomy specimens. An attempt has been made to include photomicrographs showing the more usual appearances as well as some of the unusual patterns encountered in most common lesions of the breast. In addition some of the rarer forms of mammary pathology have been illustrated, sometimes extensively, where this was considered important in the differential diagnosis and where photomicrographs of good quality were available. Some of the low power photomicrographs lack detail but have been retained as they illustrate important microanatomical or architectural patterns. The majority of the photomicrographs are of histological preparations stained with haematoxylin and eosin, but a few special stains have been used to illustrate certain specific features. Only occasional photographs of gross specimens have been included. This is not to belittle the importance of gross appearances: indeed microscopic examination of any tissue should always be complemented by careful naked-eye examination. A few mammographic pictures have also been included to illustrate characteristic patterns. There are no photomicrographs of cytological preparations as these were considered outside the scope of this book and excellent atlases of mammary cytology already exist. It is hoped that this atlas will prove useful to surgical pathologists and others interested in the histological appearances of the breast. It is not intended as a comprehensive study of breast diseases, and details of clinical presentation and treatment have only been mentioned briefly.

Acknowledgements

I would like to express my thanks to all the staff at the Hedley Atkins Unit, New Cross Hospital, for their help in the preparation of this atlas. The manuscript was typed by Susan Richardson and Patricia Merrony with assistance from Alice Rainger and Rita McLaren and technical help with the word processor from Ken Miller. Many of the photomicrographs are of sections prepared by Marian Egan and Ken Miller and Ken also took several of the gross photographs. Other photomicrographs are of sections prepared at the Royal Marsden Hospital, London by David Kellock and his colleagues. All the clinical and mammographic photographs and some of the gross photographs also come from the Royal Marsden Hospital and were prepared by Kenneth Moreman and Milena Potucek.

In addition to the above I am particularly indebted to Professor Noel Gowing for his help with all aspects of this atlas. Without his continued assistance and encouragement it would never have been completed. I am also grateful to Wolfe Medical Publications Limited for permission to use some of the illustrations from *A Colour Atlas of Tumour Histopathology* by Professor N. F. C. Gowing.

Accurate histological diagnosis can only be made if the specimen has been adequately sampled. Blocks of tissue for histological examination should include areas of obviously gross abnormality as well as representative samples of all the submitted tissue. *In situ* carcinoma, particularly of the lobular type, is often not discernible on gross examination, and infiltrating carcinoma can sometimes be difficult to detect macroscopically, particularly when the tumour is very diffuse with little productive fibrosis. Such tumours can often be felt more easily than they can be seen. Even when an obviously benign lesion is found on gross examination the surrounding tissue should always be sampled.

Tissue biopsied on the basis of an abnormal mammogram, in the absence of physical findings, merits particular attention. Specimen radiographs must be compared with the preoperative mammogram to confirm that the lesional tissue has been removed. This is particularly useful in locating calcification, but may not be so helpful in identifying mammographically suspicious areas which do not contain calcium deposits. The specimen radiograph should also be used by the pathologist as a guide to localizing the suspicious area when selecting blocks; further radiographs of the sliced tissue may be particularly helpful for this purpose. Calcification should be identified not only in the tissue blocks but also in the histology sections. Furthermore, it should be realized that carcinoma is sometimes found in non-calcified tissue immediately adjacent to an area of benign calcification.

The need for careful, thorough gross examination also applies to mastectomy specimens. Multifocal carcinoma may be identified and the overall appearance of the remaining breast should be examined, both macroscopically and microscopically, to further knowledge and understanding of the relationship of

Table 1 Classification of mammary carcinoma

Tumour type	Approximate % of different types
IN SITU CARCINOMA	
In situ duct carcinoma (with or without Paget's disease of the nipple; including intracystic carcinoma)	5
In situ lobular carcinoma	3
INFILTRATING CARCINOMA	
Infiltrating duct carcinoma Without special features or not otherwise specified (NOS) (with prominent desmoplasia (scirrhous pattern) or without prominent desmoplasia; with or without prominent intraduct carcinoma; with or without Paget's disease of the nipple) With special features	72
Medullary carcinoma with lymphoid stroma	3
Mucoid carcinoma	2
Tubular carcinoma	2
Infiltrating lobular carcinoma	12
Rare varieties of mammary carcinoma Carcinoid tumour of breast Signet-ring cell carcinoma Secretory or juvenile carcinoma Adenoid cystic carcinoma Squamous cell carcinoma Spindle cell (pseudosarcomatous) carcinoma Carcinoma with cartilaginous or osseous metaplasia Apocrine carcinoma	1
CARCINOMAS WITH PARTICULAR CLINICAL MANIFESTATIONS Paget's disease of the nipple Inflammatory carcinoma	

mammary carcinoma to other pathological changes within the breast tissue. Careful identification and dissection of axillary lymph nodes is important in order to establish the number and extent of involved nodes, as well as other features of prognostic significance such as the extranodal extension of metastases.

Adequate fixation and processing of specimens is always important, but samples of mammary tissue need particular attention. Histological interpretation of some lesions can be extremely difficult in inadequately prepared tissue.

The histological interpretation of most breast biopsies presents no problem, but occasionally mammary lesions can provide some of the most difficult differential diagnoses encountered by the surgical pathologist. Close co-operation between clinician and pathologist is particularly important in this field. Care should always be taken to ensure that the pathological findings correlate with and explain the clinical and mammographic features. If no cause for the clinical abnormality, such as a nipple discharge, is found, even after extensive sampling of the biopsy specimen, this should be recorded. It is always possible that the lesional tissue has not been removed. Conversely, it is equally important to realize that cyclical changes in the epithelium and stroma of the normal breast can produce clinical nodularity or a mass leading to biopsy. Pathologists should not hesitate to report the presence of normal breast tissue in a specimen. In the past many normal biopsies have been labelled as fibrocystic disease or fibroadenosis, for it was considered that there must be some pathological explanation for all clinical abnormalities.

Classification of Mammary Carcinoma

The classification of mammary carcinoma remains somewhat controversial. The system used in this atlas (Table 1) is based on both histogenetic and morphologic considerations and adopts the two major criteria which are used in most classifications, namely the presence or absence of invasion, and the origin, from either ducts or lobules. Although the second criterion was originally considered to be strictly anatomical, it is now generally accepted that nearly all mammary carcinomas arise from the terminal ductal lobular unit, and the concept that lobular carcinomas only arise from the lobules and duct carcinoma from the more proximal ducts is an oversimplification. There is probably considerable overlap, and the terms 'duct' and 'lobular' are now used to refer to the histological and cytological appearances of the neoplasm rather than to the actual site of origin. The great majority of mammary carcinomas are of the infiltrating duct type and further division of this group is based on morphological features as seen both macroscopically and microscopically. The classification of all mammary neoplasms adopted in this atlas differs in only minor details from that promulgated by the World Health Organization[1].

Selection of blocks of tissue for histological examination should always include both the periphery and centre of the tumour. Mixed carcinomas displaying two or more different types are not unusual and only by adequate sampling can their true nature be assessed. Even then the occasional carcinoma is extremely difficult to classify and indeed it is not always possible to distinguish between tumours of duct and lobular type.

The relative incidence of different types of carcinoma appears to vary with the geographical area and also with the circumstances of diagnosis: for example, patients presenting to a screening clinic versus those referred to the outpatient department of a general hospital. The figures given here are based on the latter population of patients.

Reference

1. World Health Organization, Geneva, Switzerland (1982). Histological typing of breast tumours. *Tumori,* **68**, 181

The Normal Breast

2

The structure of the normal, mature, resting female breast is shown in Figures 2.1–2.7. The epithelial component, which comprises only a very small proportion of the total volume of the breast, is found mainly in the upper outer quadrant and central area. Most of the breast is composed of supporting fibrous tissue and fat. In the prepubertal breast the epithelial component consists of ducts without lobules. Several years before puberty lactiferous ducts begin to grow and branch. At the time of menarche the lobules begin to develop and these are the potentially milk-producing part of the glands.

The normal resting lobule is seen in Figures 2.1 and 2.2, and comprises a group of small blind ending units variously known as acini, alveoli or terminal ductules[1]. These drain into a small ductule (sometimes known as the terminal duct). This terminal ductal lobular unit[2] is surrounded by loose vascular connective tissue containing fibroblasts and a few lymphocytes. The intralobular connective tissue is easily distinguishable from the denser interlobular connective tissue. Each ductule drains from the lobule via larger ducts to a segmental duct. The duct system of each segment of the breast leads to a dilated lactiferous sinus beneath the nipple (Figures 2.3 and 2.4). From the lactiferous sinus a collecting duct extends to the nipple surface. About ten collecting ducts open onto the nipple and in the resting breast they are normally plugged with keratin. Numerous sebaceous and apocrine glands are also found in the nipple. The former are illustrated in Figure 2.5, in which the erectile muscle of the nipple can also be seen. Because of the very irregular outline of the lactiferous sinus, tangential cutting may produce the appearance of invaginations, which can be mistaken for a papilloma or epithelial hyperplasia.

Throughout the breast the glandular tissue consists of a double layer of epithelial cells (Figure 2.6). The inner layer is composed of columnar or cuboidal epithelium. The outer layer consists of myoepithelium which can be clearly demonstrated by staining unfixed frozen sections for alkaline phosphatase, an enzyme present in high concentration in the cytoplasm of the myoepithelial cells (Figure 2.7). In formalin-fixed paraffin-embedded tissue actin and myosin, present in myoepithelial cells, can be demonstrated using immunohistochemical techniques. The mammary ducts are surrounded by a layer of elastic fibres, but this does not extend into the lobules. The amount of elastic tissue increases with age and parity[1].

The changes which occur in the breast during pregnancy and lactation are shown in Figures 2.8 and 2.9. There is marked proliferation of the glandular tissue, with an increase both in the number of lobules and in the number of acini within each lobule. The cells lining these units exhibit evidence of secretory activity. Following cessation of lactation there is involution of the lobular elements. Even in the resting breast some lobules are better developed than others, and although nowhere near as markedly as in the lactating breast, the epithelium may show evidence of secretory activity[3]. This is possibly related to the menstrual cycle, although there is disagreement in the literature concerning correlation of the presence of secretions with the stage of the cycle[4]. Recent studies have also shown that the number of mitoses in the lobular epithelium and the number of cells undergoing apoptosis are related to the stage of the menstrual cycle[5]. Inactive lobules have fewer acini, and a denser stroma.

After the menopause most of the lobules regress to an inactive pattern, and eventually there is loss of much of the glandular tissue, particularly the lobules including their specialized stroma. The breast of an elderly woman is demonstrated in Figures 2.10 and 2.11, and consists mainly of fatty tissue with only a few residual ducts and vessels. Occasionally there is persistence of lobules in the postmenopausal breast and there is some evidence to suggest that this is associated with an increased incidence of carcinoma[3]. Involution can also result in cyst formation by fusion of acini. This cystic lobular involution (Figure 2.12) is sometimes mistaken for cystic disease[1].

The normal male breast is shown in Chapter 8. The appearance is similar to that of the prepubertal female breast and the glandular tissue consists of only ducts with no lobules.

References

1. Azzopardi, J. G. (1979). *Problems in Breast Pathology*, p. 8. (Vol. 11 in Bennington, J. L. (consulting ed.) *Major Problems in Pathology*.) (London, Philadelphia and Toronto: Saunders)

2. Wellings, S. R., Jensen, H. M. and Marcum, R. G. (1975). An atlas of subgross pathology of the human breast with special reference to possible precancerous lesions. *J. Natl. Cancer Inst.*, **55**, 231

3. Jensen, H. M. (1981). Breast pathology emphasising pre-cancerous and cancer-associated lesions. In Bulbrook, R. D. and Taylor, D. J. (eds.) *Commentaries on Research in Breast Disease*, Vol. 2, p. 41. (New York: Liss)

4. Vogel, P. M., Georgiade, N. G., Fetter, B. F., Vogel, F. S. and McCarty, K. S. Jr. (1981). The correlation of histologic changes in the human breast with the menstrual cycle. *Am. J. Pathol.*, **104**, 23

5. Anderson, T. J., Ferguson, D. J. P. and Raab, G. M. (1982). Cell turnover in the 'resting' human breast: influence of parity, contraceptive pill, age and laterality. *Br. J. Cancer*, **46**, 376

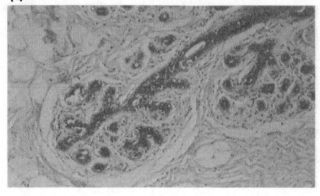

Figure 2.1. Normal breast. Section showing two lobules with a duct leading away from one. The intralobular stroma is looser and more cellular than the interlobular stroma; the latter is composed of mature fibrous tissue and adipose tissue in varying proportions.   H & E × 96

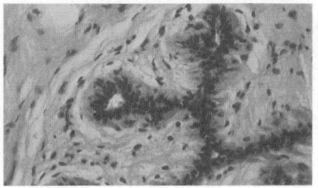

Figure 2.2 Normal breast. Part of a normal lobule at higher magnification. The loose cellular stroma within the lobule contrasts with the surrounding interlobular stroma at the top left-hand corner of the field. The acini and ductules have a double cell layer: cells immediately adjacent to the lumen, and an outer mantle of myoepithelial cells. In this photomicrograph, the cytoplasm of the myoepithelial cells is stained brightly with eosin.   H & E × 240

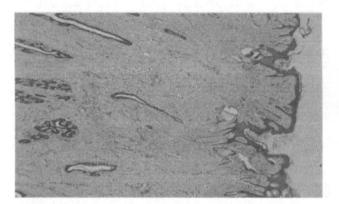

Figure 2.3 Normal nipple. Section showing large lactiferous ducts, cut in various planes, converging towards the surface. The skin is covered by an epidermal layer, with associated sebaceous glands but no hair follicles. H & E × 24

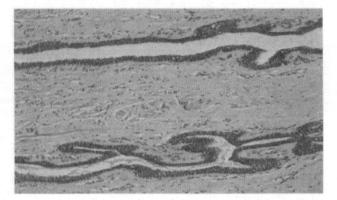

Figure 2.4 Normal nipple. Two lactiferous ducts are shown in longitudinal section. In some parts of the field the double cell layer is apparent, the outer row of nuclei being those of the myoepithelial mantle. The apparent infolding seen in the lower duct results from the particular plane of section passing through a zone of mild tortuosity; it must not be confused with a true papillary ingrowth.   H & E × 96

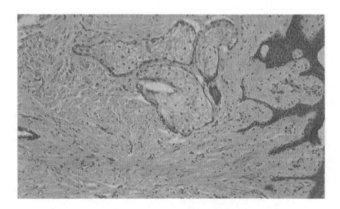

Figure 2.5 Normal nipple. Higher magnification of the section illustrated in Figure 2.3 showing the epidermis with subjacent sebaceous gland, and smooth muscle fibres mingled with the dermal collagen.   H & E × 96

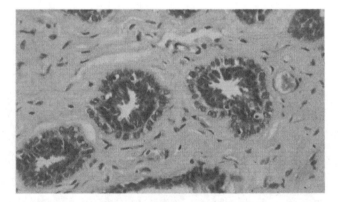

Figure 2.6 Normal breast. Section showing several ducts cut transversely and displaying very clearly the double cell layers.   H & E × 240

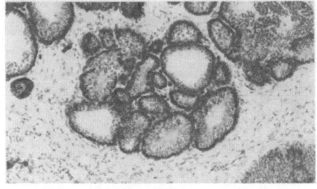

Figure 2.7 Myoepithelial cells surrounding mammary ducts. A fresh unfixed section stained for alkaline phosphatase. The myoepithelial cells stain red because of their high enzyme content. They form regular mantles around the ducts. Azo coupling technique for alkaline phosphatase × 96

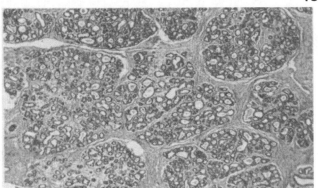

Figure 2.8 Pregnancy changes in breast. Hyperplasia has resulted in crowding together of the lobules. The ductules are somewhat dilated and contain eosinophilic secretion. H & E × 24

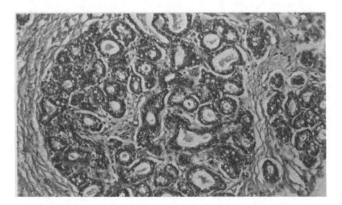

Figure 2.9 Pregnancy changes in breast. Higher magnification of the section illustrated in the previous figure. The acinar cells have vacuolated cytoplasm indicative of their secretory activity. H & E × 96

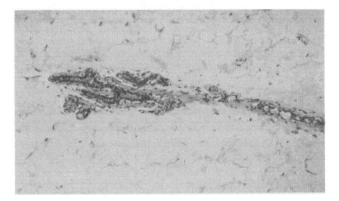

Figure 2.10 Atrophic changes in breast of elderly woman. Section from the breast of an elderly woman. A duct has been cut longitudinally and runs horizontally across the field; it originates in a lobule which displays marked atrophy with loss of both acini and of the specialized intralobular connective tissue stroma. The interlobular stroma is predominantly fatty. H & E × 96

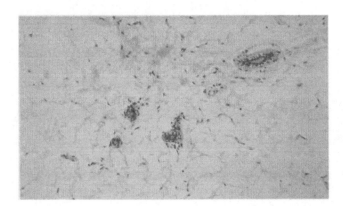

Figure 2.11 Atrophic changes in breast of elderly woman. The mammary parenchyma comprises a few small widely scattered ducts in a predominantly fatty stroma. H & E × 96

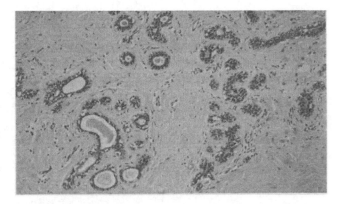

Figure 2.12 Cystic lobular atrophy of the breast. The normal lobular architecture is much distorted as a result of a decrease in the number of acini, and dilatation and fusion of the residual acini. H & E × 96

Inflammatory Lesions

3

Inflammatory lesions of the breast are not common and are rarely submitted to the histopathologist for diagnosis. Acute inflammation in the form of an abscess is most often seen during lactation. Occasionally a chronic abscess of the breast is drained and a biopsy may be taken from its walls. Tissue may also be taken from a chronic mammary fistula. Inflammatory tissue from these sites shows no particular or unusual feature. However, certain specific inflammatory lesions of the breast are occasionally encountered.

Tuberculosis

Tuberculosis of the breast is very rare in Western countries, and is infrequent even in those parts of the world where tuberculosis is a common disease. It usually occurs in women between 20 and 40 years of age; pregnancy and lactation are thought to increase susceptibility to tuberculous mastitis[1,2]. However many cases have been described in older women and occasional cases in men[3]. Clinically the disease may present as one or more nodules eventually progressing to chronic discharging sinuses. In elderly women fibrosis is often the dominant feature. This may involve the entire breast and differentiation from mammary carcinoma can be extremely difficult. Histological examination shows the typical caseating granulomas composed of histiocytes and Langhans' giant cells (Figures 3.1 and 3.2). Acid-fast bacilli are usually very sparse and often cannot be found in histological sections, although their demonstration is clearly a valuable confirmation of the diagnosis. The mammary lesion may be secondary to widespread infection but in over half the cases the infection appears to be confined to the breast without evidence of tuberculosis elsewhere[1]. Although some enlargment of the axillary lymph node is present in about 50% of cases, caseous lymphadenitis is uncommon.

Mycotic, Parasitic and Other Miscellaneous Inflammatory Lesions of the Breast

Various fungal diseases of the breast have been reported, including cryptococcosis, blastomycosis, histoplasmosis and actinomycosis[4,5]. Rare cases of filariasis, echinococcosis and cysticercosis have also been recorded[4,6]. Lymph nodes are occasionally found within the anatomical confines of the breast, and such ectopic nodes may be involved in a variety of non-specific and specific reactive and inflammatory processes, such as toxoplasmosis (Figure 3.3).

Sarcoidosis

In this disease, involvement of the breast is rare, but has been reported in patients with generalized sarcoidosis.

Granulomatous Mastitis

Apart from the granulomatous breast lesions mentioned above, there is the rare and puzzling condition called granulomatous mastitis by Kessler and Wolloch[7]. Figures 3.4 and 3.5 show the typical histological appearances in which the granulomatous inflammation is confined to the lobules. The granulomas are usually non-caseous and are composed of histiocytes and multinucleated giant cells, of both the foreign-body and Langhans' types; neutrophils are often present. This lesion usually occurs in parous women of child-bearing age and is frequently diagnosed clinically as carcinoma. Differentiation from duct ectasia, fat necrosis and cyst rupture should be possible on histological examination but tuberculosis, mycotic infection and sarcoidosis must also be excluded. Although granulomatous mastitis may be due to an infective agent, none has been identified to date and the possibility of an immunological aetiology has been suggested[7,8].

Cyst Rupture

This condition, illustrated in Figures 3.6 and 3.7, results from the rupture of a tension cyst with leakage of the contents leading to an inflammatory reaction in the surrounding tissues. In the early stages, the inflammatory changes predominate, but later fibrosis occurs. The condition may simulate carcinoma on both clinical and pathological examination. Macroscopically, cysts are usually present in the surrounding breast, and, in the region of the rupture, patchy yellow discoloration similar to fat necrosis is often seen. In lesions of longer duration, the tissue may be extremely firm. The early infiltrate consists of lymphocytes, plasma cells and histiocytes with many foamy macrophages producing a lipogranulomatous reaction. In older lesions, there is fibroblastic proliferation. On cursory examination, both these patterns may be confused with infiltrating carcinoma, but careful study should preclude such an error. The use of elastic stains in the differentiation between duct ectasia and cyst rupture is discussed later, in Chapters 4 and 5.

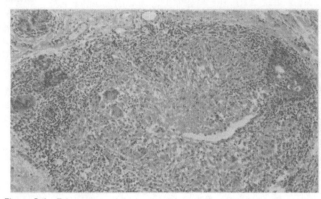

Figure 3.1 Tuberculosis of the breast. A lesion excised from the breast of a 65-year-old woman who had had osseous and genitourinary tuberculosis in the past. Mammary ductules are present on the extreme left; most of the field is occupied by a caseating granuloma, featuring epithelioid cells, giant cells and peripheral lymphocytes.   H & E × 96

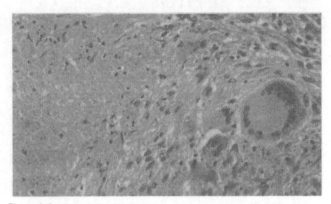

Figure 3.2 Tuberculosis of the breast. Higher magnification of the lesion illustrated in Figure 3.1, showing caseation on the left, and epithelioid cells and Langhans' giant cells on the right.   H & E × 240

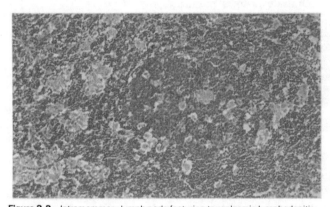

Figure 3.3 Intramammary lymph node featuring toxoplasmic lymphadenitis. Sections of a lump excised from the outer part of the breast of a young woman. Although anatomically within the breast, the lump proved to be a lymph node with microscopic features suggestive of toxoplasmosis. The diagnosis was confirmed by serology. The photomicrograph shows a prominent reaction centre in the right half of the field. Small, irregularly shaped clusters of epithelioid cells are present, both in the interfollicular pulp and within the follicle itself.   H & E × 96

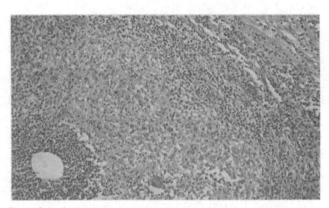

Figure 3.4 Granulomatous mastitis. The central portion of the granuloma (bottom left-hand corner) contains many neutrophil polymorphs. There is a broad zone of histiocytes with a few multinucleated cells and a peripheral band of lymphocytes.   H & E × 96

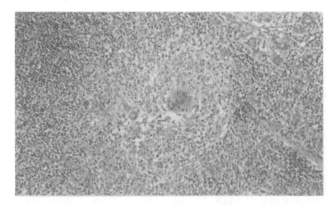

Figure 3.5 Granulomatous mastitis. Another granuloma forming part of the same lesion as that illustrated in the previous figure. Here, polymorphs are not present and there is no necrosis. The granuloma comprises a mass of histiocytes with multinucleated giant cells and a peripheral zone of lymphocytes.   H & E × 96

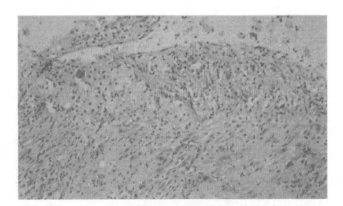

Figure 3.6 Breast cyst with destruction of epithelial lining. This section shows part of the cyst wall, the lumen being at the top of the field. The epithelium has been destroyed, and the cyst is lined by granulation tissue comprising capillary blood vessels, fibroblasts and a few inflammatory cells.   H & E × 96

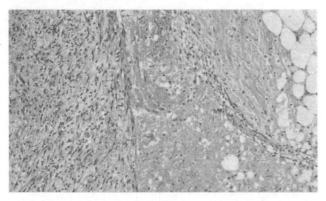

Figure 3.7 Breast cyst with destruction of epithelial lining. In this section the lumen contains amorphous eosinophilic debris and blood. The epithelium has been destroyed and the lining consists of a thick layer of granulation tissue, seen on the left of the field. H & E × 96

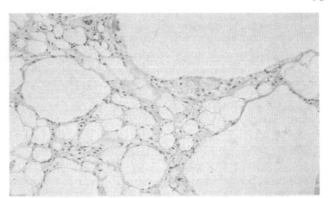

Figure 3.8 Fat necrosis. Liberation of fat from the necrotic adipose tissue has produced a collection of lipid-filled spaces of various sizes. The spaces are empty in sections of paraffin-embedded material. Between the spaces there are some histiocytes with foamy cytoplasm. H & E × 96

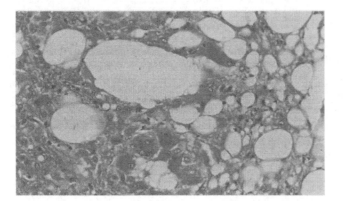

Figure 3.9 Fat necrosis. The extracellular lipid, which originally occupied the rounded empty spaces, has evoked a granulomatous response, predominantly histiocytic in this field. H & E × 240

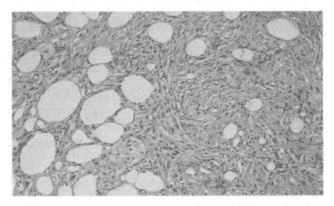

Figure 3.10 Fat necrosis. In this lesion, the lipid-filled spaces have become more widely separated as the granulomatous reaction progresses. Many of the cells are histiocytes, but there are also some spindle-shaped fibroblasts. H & E × 96

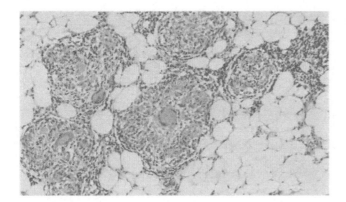

Figure 3.11 Fat necrosis. This photomicrograph shows another microscopic pattern which may develop; small, non-caseating tuberculoid granulomas, featuring epithelioid cells, Langhans' giant cells and peripheral zones of lymphocytes. H & E × 96

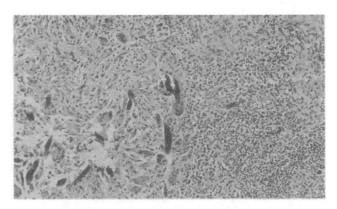

Figure 3.12 Foreign-body granuloma. A section of a breast lesion resulting from a retained swab introduced at the time of a previous biopsy. The fibres of the swab are stained red and there is a surrounding inflammatory reaction, with numerous lymphocytes, plasmacytes, histiocytes and multinucleated giant cells. Congo red × 96

Fat Necrosis

Fat necrosis in the breast, as elsewhere in the body, can produce a wide range of clinical and pathological appearances. It may simulate carcinoma both on clinical and mammographic examination, but the diagnosis is usually obvious on macroscopic and microscopic study[9]. In the gross, the bright-yellow opaque necrotic fat contrasts sharply with the surrounding translucent viable adipose tissue. On histological examination of the early lesion, the necrotic tissue consists of vacuoles of fat infiltrated by inflammatory cells, mainly lymphocytes and foamy macrophages (Figures 3.8–3.10). Multinucleate foreign-body giant cells may also be present and sometimes these appear to line small cyst-like spaces (Figure 3.11). In the later stages, there is a fibroblastic reaction and eventually fibrosis, sometimes with calcification. Granules of yellow-brown pigment are frequently present in the older lesions and appear to be a mixture of haemosiderin and lipofuscin. The histological pattern of fat necrosis must be differentiated from the changes associated with cyst rupture and duct ectasia. Examination of changes in the adjacent ducts and lobules should help to distinguish between these various conditions.

Fat necrosis is most commonly seen in obese women with pendulous breasts. It is frequently stated that there is always a history of trauma, but personal observation indicates that this can only be elicited in about half the patients.

Foreign-body Granuloma

Foreign bodies within the breast are rare – they may be introduced as the result of an accident or during surgery (Figure 3.12). Some prosthetic procedures also involve the introduction of foreign material, such as silicone, and may result in a severe reaction and disfiguration.

References

1. Cohen, C. (1977). Tuberculous mastitis. A review of 34 cases. *S. Afr. Med. J.*, **52**, 12

2. Ikard, R. W. and Perkins, D. (1977). Mammary tuberculosis: a rare modern disease. *South. Med. J.*, **70**, 208

3. Tabar, L., Kett, K. and Nemeth, A. (1976). Tuberculosis of the breast. *Radiology*, **118**, 587

4. Symmers, W.St.C. (1978). The breasts. In Symmers, W.St.C. (ed.) *Systemic Pathology*, 2nd Edn., Vol. 4, Chap. 28, p. 1760. (Edinburgh, London and New York: Churchill Livingstone)

5. Salfelder, K. and Schwarz, J. (1975). Mycotic 'pseudo tumors' of the breast. Report of four cases. *Arch. Surg.*, **110**, 751

6. Chandrasoma, P. T. and Mendis, K. N. (1978). Filarial infection of the breast. *Am. J. Trop. Med. Hyg.*, **27**, 770

7. Kessler, E. and Wolloch, Y. (1972). Granulomatous mastitis: A lesion clinically simulating carcinoma. *Am. J. Clin. Pathol.*, **58**, 642

8. Fletcher, A., Magrath, I. M., Riddell, R. H. and Talbot, I. C. (1982). Granulomatous mastitis: a report of seven cases. *J. Clin. Pathol.*, **35**, 941

9. Meyer, J. E., Silverman, P. and Gandbhir, L. (1978). Fat necrosis of the breast. *Arch. Surg.*, **113**, 801

Duct Ectasia

Many names have been applied to this condition, including periductal mastitis, plasma cell mastitis, comedo mastitis and mastitis obliterans, but the term 'mammary duct ectasia' suggested by Haagensen[1] in 1951 is perhaps the most commonly used. Although this condition may occur in women under 45 years of age it is more usually seen in older women[1,2]. In postmortem studies, duct ectasia is found quite frequently in postmenopausal women – even in those who had no symptoms during life[3]. The aetiology of duct ectasia remains obscure and, although it is more commonly seen in parous than in nulliparous women, the exact relationship to pregnancy and lactation is not clear[2,4].

Clinically, duct ectasia may be impossible to differentiate from a carcinoma. Nipple retraction and nipple discharge, which may be bloodstained, are frequent. Subareolar thickening may be present and pain and tenderness in the subareolar region are not uncommon. On gross examination of the tissue dilated ducts containing green and brown tenacious fluid or paste-like material are often seen. In the late stages of the disease, however, there is marked fibrosis and no distinctive macroscopic appearance may be demonstrated. The condition usually begins beneath the nipple and may then spread to affect the smaller ducts, often involving only one mammary segment. It has been claimed that the condition frequently passes unrecognized by pathologists who confuse it with cystic disease or fat necrosis[5]. The histological features of duct ectasia vary considerably with the phase of the disease. The various phases are illustrated in Figures 4.1–4.12. There is disagreement as to whether inflammatory changes precede dilatation of the ducts in the early stages of the disease, or whether dilatation occurs first and the inflammatory process is secondary to stagnation of the duct contents and subsequent leakage into the surrounding tissue[4,5]. In the fully developed lesion the ducts are dilated, filled with amorphous debris, and display periductal fibrosis and inflammatory cell infiltration. Patchy hyperplasia of the epithelium may be present, but more often the epithelial lining is attenuated and may be replaced by granulation tissue containing foreign-body giant cells and foamy macrophages. In the well-developed lesion there is patchy destruction of the elastic fibres of the duct wall, and Azzopardi[5] has suggested that demonstration of patches of elastic fibres around the dilated ducts is an invaluable diagnostic feature in distinguishing duct ectasia from cystic disease, since elastic fibres are absent around mammary cysts. In some cases the lumen of the duct is totally obliterated, first by granulation tissue and later by fibrosis. When obliteration occurs, proliferation of the epithelium may produce a collarette of small epithelial-lined spaces at the periphery of the original duct. Calcification may occur in duct ectasia either in the lumen or in the walls (Figures 4.10 and 4.11). In the latter situation it may be deposited in a ring-like fashion which gives rise to a characteristic appearance on mammography illustrated in Figure 4.12. The nipple retraction frequently seen in the late stage of the disease is probably due to contraction of the fibrous tissue around the ducts[4].

References

1. Haagensen, C. D. (1951). Mammary-duct ectasia. A disease that may simulate carcinoma. *Cancer*, **4**, 749

2. Walker, J. C. and Sandison, A. T. (1964). Mammary-duct ectasia. A clinical study. *Br. J. Surg.*, **51**, 350

3. Sandison, A. T. (1962). *An Autopsy Study of the Adult Human Breast*. (National Cancer Institute Monograph No. 8.) (Washington DC: US Department of Health, Education and Welfare)

4. Rees, B. I., Gravelle, I. H. and Hughes, L. E. (1977). Nipple retraction in duct ectasia. *Br. J. Surg.*, **64**, 577

5. Azzopardi, J. G. (1979). *Problems in Breast Pathology*, p. 57. (Vol. 11 in Bennington, J. L. (consulting ed.) *Major Problems in Pathology*.) (London, Philadelphia and Toronto: Saunders)

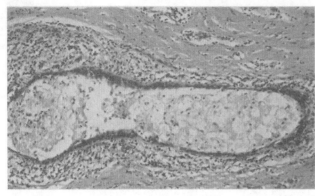

Figure 4.1 Mammary duct ectasia. The duct is moderately dilated and is surrounded by a mantle of inflammatory cells, predominantly lymphocytes and histiocytes. The lumen contains many cells with abundant, foamy cytoplasm. This is an early lesion, and periductal sclerosis has not developed. H & E × 96

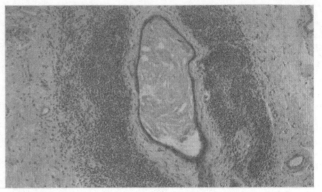

Figure 4.2 Mammary duct ectasia. This photomicrograph illustrates a more advanced stage of the disease process. The duct is dilated, containing eosinophilic proteinaceous coagulum, the wall is thickened by fibrosis and there is a broad corona of lymphocytes and plasmacytes. H & E × 96

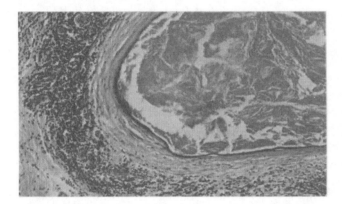

Figure 4.3 Mammary duct ectasia. The dilated duct is lined by a flattened layer of nondescript epithelial cells. The lumen contains amorphous eosinophilic material. The wall is thickened by dense fibrosis, and there is a surrounding mantle of chronic inflammatory cells. H & E × 96

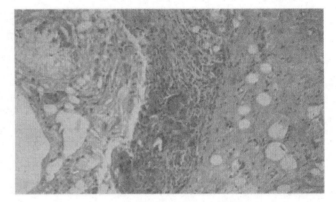

Figure 4.4 Mammary duct ectasia. In this section the duct epithelium has been completely destroyed and is replaced by granulation tissue comprising histiocytes and multinucleated giant cells of foreign-body type. The lumen (on the left) contains amorphous eosinophilic debris and a few degenerate cells with pyknotic nuclei. H & E × 96

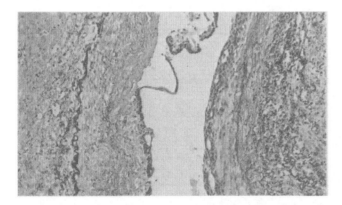

Figure 4.5 Mammary duct ectasia. Section stained for elastic fibres. The lumen of the duct runs vertically across the centre of the photomicrograph. On the left, the elastic lamina is virtually intact, and there is fibrous thickening of the wall beneath it. To the right of the lumen, fibrosis has resulted in destruction of the normal pattern, with fragmentation of the elastic fibres. Orcein elastic stain × 96

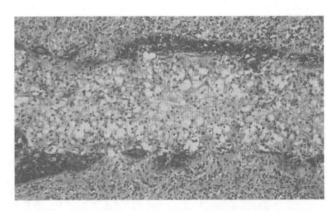

Figure 4.6 Mammary duct ectasia. In this example there is marked periductal mastitis, with focal disruption of the duct wall and penetration of the epithelium by inflammatory cells. The photomicrograph shows part of the duct cut longitudinally and running transversely across the field. H & E × 96

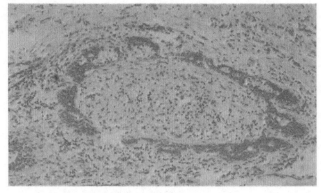

Figure 4.7 Mammary duct ectasia, proceeding to luminal obliteration. Following the penetration of the duct wall by granulation tissue, organization of the luminal contents is taking place. The lumen contains lymphocytes, histiocytes and fibroblasts. The epithelium has partially regenerated to form imperfect tubular structures. H & E × 96

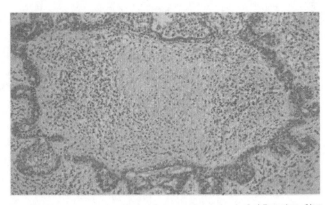

Figure 4.8 Mammary duct ectasia, proceeding to luminal obliteration. This section shows a more advanced stage of the process. Apart from inflammatory cells, the lumen contains some palely-eosinophilic collagen. Again, regeneration of the epithelium has produced a ring of small tubular structures. H & E × 96

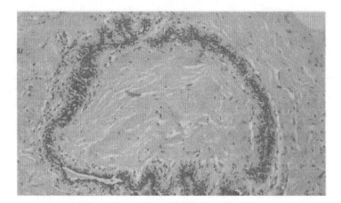

Figure 4.9 Mammary duct ectasia, with luminal obliteration. Here the process of organization of the luminal contents has been completed. The original lumen is replaced by a mass of mature collagenous tissue and regenerative proliferation of the epithelium has produced a collarette of small tubules encircling the original perimeter of the duct. H & E × 96

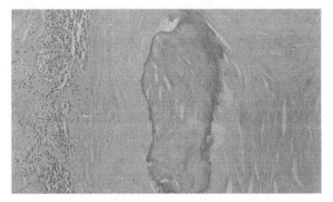

Figure 4.10 Mammary duct ectasia, with luminal obliteration and calcification. The space originally occupied by the duct lumen is now filled by dense, sparsely cellular fibrous tissue. The central part of the fibrous tissue mass is calcified, as indicated by the bluish staining with haematoxylin. On the left there is a residual, periductal lymphocytic infiltrate. H & E × 96

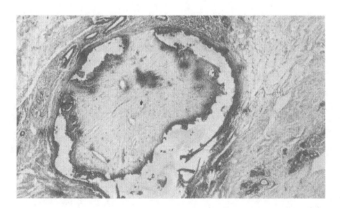

Figure 4.11 Mammary duct ectasia, with luminal obliteration and calcification. As in the previous section, the lumen has been replaced by a dense, sparsely cellular mass of collagen. In this example the calcium, stained blue with haematoxylin, has been laid down in an annular configuration. Owing to the friability of the tissue, artefactual crushing and clefting have occurred in the section. H & E × 96

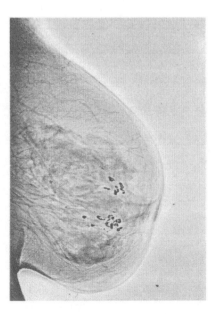

Figure 4.12 Xeromammogram with calcification in mammary duct ectasia. Xeromammogram showing coarse calcification with tubular, rounded and ring-like forms typical of calcification in ectatic ducts.

Although some non-neoplastic lesions of the breast form distinct entities, the majority show a wide variety of proliferative and regressive changes in the glandular tissues and stroma. There has been much discussion concerning the best designation for this heterogenous group of benign breast lesions; terms such as benign mastopathy, mammary dysplasia, fibroadenosis and fibrocystic disease have been used. The term 'mammary dysplasia' has been criticized on the ground that dysplasia has a connotation of premalignancy when applied to other organs, such as the cervix uteri. 'Fibrocystic disease' and 'fibroadenosis' tend to suggest specific changes which may or may not be present. Azzopardi[1] recommended the term 'cystic disease' when only cysts are present and 'cystic hyperplasia' when, as is more usual, there is accompanying epithelial hyperplasia. These terms indicate both the commonest (cystic) and the most important (hyperplastic) changes.

Whether all biopsies labelled as cystic disease or cystic hyperplasia really represent pathological changes in the breast is debatable. Many of the features traditionally included under this heading – such as cysts, adenosis, apocrine metaplasia and epithelial hyperplasia – are seen in autopsy studies in a very high proportion of breasts from women without clinical disease. It may well be that the diference between normal breasts and those with clinical features of disease leading to biopsy are differences of degree rather than of quality[2].

Epithelial Hyperplasia

Epithelial hyperplasia can affect any part of the duct or lobular system but nearly always involves the terminal ductal lobular unit and is rarely seen in larger ducts. There is considerable variation in both the quantity and the pattern. Although the condition is generally divided into ductal and lobular hyperplasia, the subgross sections of Wellings and co-workers[3] suggest that the hyperplasia nearly always involves the lobule, and they refer to the two patterns as 'atypical lobule type A', with the coarser ductular pattern, and 'atypical lobule type B', in which the lobular microarchitecture is retained. In common with other authorities[4] Wellings et al[3] grade the changes according to the amount of hyperplasia and the degree of cellular atypia, claiming that there is a direct progression from epithelial hyperplasia to carcinoma in situ. Differentiation from in situ duct or lobular carcinoma is sometimes extremely difficult. The general pattern of the lesion should be taken into account as well as the cellular detail. Benign epithelial hyperplasia is frequently accompanied by other changes of the cystic disease complex, such as cysts, apocrine metaplasia (pink cell change), columnar cell metaplasia, sclerosing adenosis and small peripheral intraduct papillomas. Areas of pink cell metaplasia often occur within the areas of epithelial hyperplasia. The overall appearance of benign hyperplasia is thus generally more complex than in situ carcinoma, which tends to display a more uniform pattern. However, it must always be remembered that carcinoma of any type can occur in association with benign changes.

Ductal Hyperplasia (Epitheliosis, Papillomatosis)

Most problems appear to arise in distinguishing ductal hyperplasia from in situ duct carcinoma. Benign epithelial proliferation results in the piling up of cells to produce irregular protrusions of varying thickness into the duct, often with complete obliteration of the lumen (Figures 5.1–5.3). The proliferating cells have irregularly shaped nuclei including spindle forms. Some of the cells appear elongated and are often arranged with parallel orientation of their long axes resulting in a 'streaming' pattern (Figure 5.4). Staining for alkaline phosphatase shows many of these cells to be myoepithelial (Figure 5.5). The cytoplasm is homogenous and cell borders indistinct; nuclei are unevenly distributed, nucleoli are inconspicuous and mitotic figures few.

Irregular spaces are frequently present within the proliferating sheets of cells and may be so numerous as to produce a pseudopapillary pattern sometimes termed papillomatosis (Figure 5.6). There can also be more regular rounded spaces lined by cells orientated towards the lumen to produce a pseudoglandular pattern (Figure 5.7). A spurious cribriform pattern may result from oedematous swelling of the stroma (Figures 5.8 and 5.9). All of these must be distinguished from cribriform intraduct carcinoma (Figure 5.10). Pink cell metaplasia may occur within areas of benign hyperplasia (Figure 5.11) and areas composed entirely of apocrine cells, sometimes demonstrating papillary infolding and a cribriform pattern, may be present (Figures 5.12 and 5.13).

Foam cells are often present within the lumen or amongst the proliferating cells of benign epithelial hyperplasia but are seen less frequently in carcinoma (Figure 5.14). Necrosis and haemorrhage on the other hand are rare in benign hyperplasia and, if they are present, care should be taken to exclude carcinoma. Foci of calcification are seen in both benign hyperplasia and in carcinoma in situ, although they are less common in the benign lesions and according to Azzopardi[1] calcific spherules and psammoma bodies hardly ever occur in benign hyperplasia.

In benign hyperplasia the myoepithelial cells often participate in the hyperplastic process, as mentioned

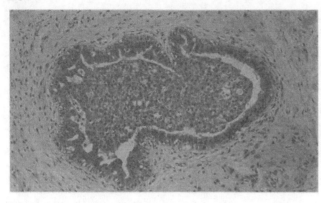

Figure 5.1 Cystic hyperplasia. This section illustrates a pattern of benign epithelial proliferation, in which the lumen of a small cyst is occupied by a solid mass of epithelial cells, attached to the lining layer at several points. H & E × 96

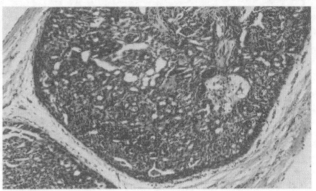

Figure 5.2 Cystic hyperplasia. Marked epithelial hyperplasia has produced an almost solid mass of cells filling and distending the lumen of the duct. H & E × 96

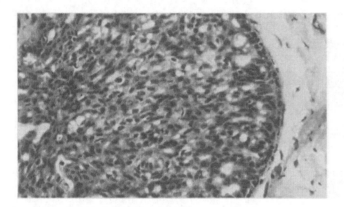

Figure 5.3 Cystic hyperplasia. Higher magnification of the lesion shown in Figure 5.2. The cell content is polymorphic: there are many fusiform cells, probably of myoepithelial type. H & E × 240

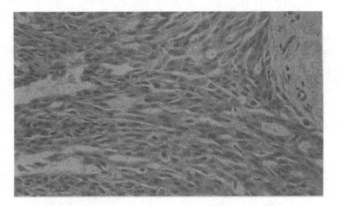

Figure 5.4 Cystic hyperplasia. An example of cystic hyperplasia in which some of the proliferating cells are spindle shaped and have eosinophilic cytoplasm; such cells are probably of myoepithelial origin. H & E × 240

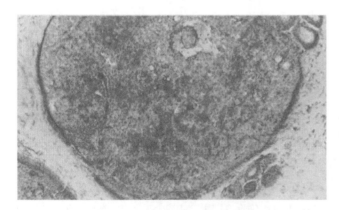

Figure 5.5 Cystic hyperplasia. The lumen of the distended duct is filled with a solid mass of epithelial cells. In this benign hyperplasia both the juxtaluminal cells and myoepithelium participate, as shown by the presence of numerous myoepithelial cells with red-staining cytoplasm (high alkaline phosphatase content). Azo coupling technique for alkaline phosphatase × 96

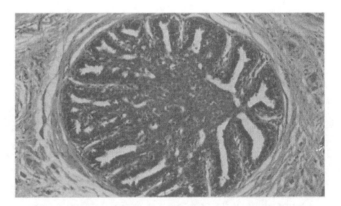

Figure 5.6 Cystic hyperplasia. In this lesion, epithelial proliferation has produced a picture reminiscent of the 'cartwheel' pattern seen in some cases of intraduct carcinoma. However, in this example, the 'spokes' have connective tissue cores and are covered by double cell layers of epithelium (juxtaluminal and myoepithelial components). Centrally there is a solid mass of irregularly arranged cells. H & E × 96

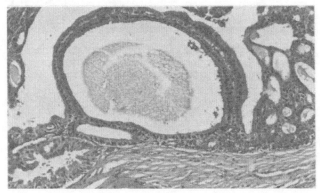

Figure 5.7   Cystic hyperplasia. Section showing part of a cyst wall, with pro-liferated epithelium forming a large intraluminal loop. In contrast to the loops seen in intraduct carcinoma, this benign lesion features pink cell metaplasia, regular orientation of the cells with their long axes disposed radially, and two discrete cell layers with intervening stroma forming the loop.   H & E × 96

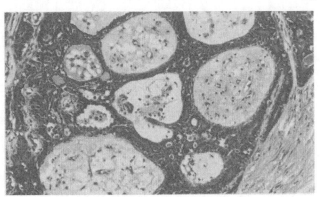

Figure 5.8   Cystic hyperplasia. In this section, there are spurious cribriform spaces, formed by oedematous connective tissue stroma containing capillary blood vessels, foamy histiocytes and a few lymphocytes.   H & E × 96

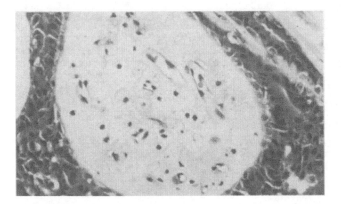

Figure 5.9   Cystic hyperplasia. Higher magnification of the section illustrated in Figure 5.8 showing one of the 'spaces' containing oedematous connective tissue with capillary blood vessels and foamy histiocytes.   H & E × 240

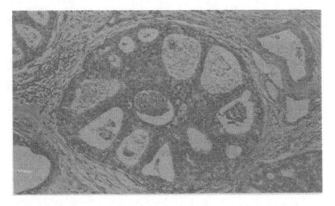
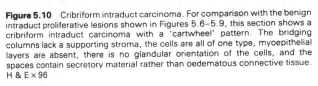

Figure 5.10   Cribriform intraduct carcinoma. For comparison with the benign intraduct proliferative lesions shown in Figures 5.6–5.9, this section shows a cribriform intraduct carcinoma with a 'cartwheel' pattern. The bridging columns lack a supporting stroma, the cells are all of one type, myoepithelial layers are absent, there is no glandular orientation of the cells, and the spaces contain secretory material rather than oedematous connective tissue. H & E × 96

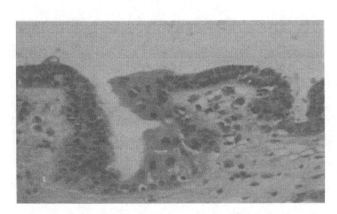

Figure 5.11   Cystic hyperplasia with pink cell metaplasia. Part of a cyst wall showing localized pink cell metaplasia affecting a group of cells interposed between unaltered epithelium.   H & E × 240

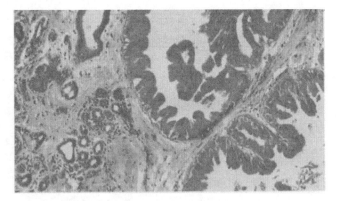

Figure 5.12   Cystic hyperplasia with pink cell metaplasia. The two cysts in the right half of the field display prominent pink cell (apocrine) metaplasia, with papillary projections into the lumina.   H & E × 96

28

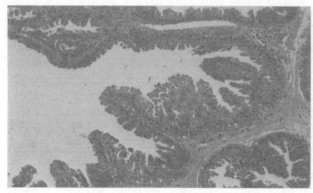

Figure 5.13 Cystic hyperplasia, with pink cell change and papillary ingrowths. In this field all the cells lining the cysts have undergone pink cell (apocrine) metaplasia and have proliferated to form papillary projections into the lumina. H & E × 96

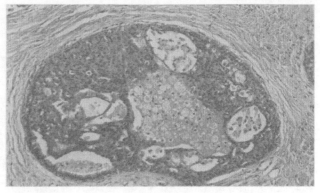

Figure 5.14 Cystic hyperplasia. Section showing a cyst whose lumen is largely occupied by epithelial cells devoid of any special arrangement. The spaces within the cellular mass are very irregular in size and shape, and many contain cells with voluminous foamy cytoplasm. H & E × 96

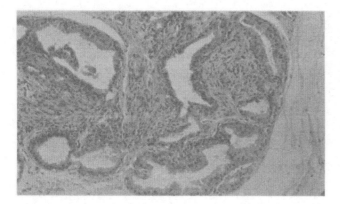

Figure 5.15 Cystic hyperplasia. Section showing pink cell metaplasia and the proliferation of spindle shaped cells of myoepithelial origin.   H & E × 96

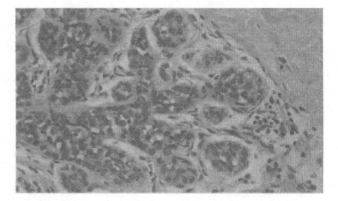

Figure 5.16 Atypical lobular hyperplasia. Part of a lobule showing mild distension of the ductules and acini by an increased number of epithelial cells. In contrast to lobular carcinoma *in situ*, nuclear aberration is inconspicuous and the cells are cohesive and do not lie loosely within dilated tubules. H & E × 240

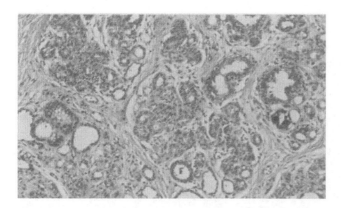

Figure 5.17 Atypical lobular hyperplasia. In this section the cells of the ductules and acini are larger than normal and have undergone proliferation, causing distortion of the lobular architecture. However, the cells are still coherent and the lumina are preserved.   H & E × 96

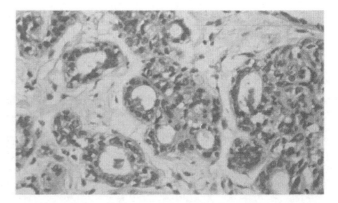

Figure 5.18 Atypical lobular hyperplasia. Higher magnification of the lesion illustrated in Figure 5.17. In contrast to lobular carcinoma *in situ*, the hyperplastic cells are coherent and the lumina are retained.   H & E × 240

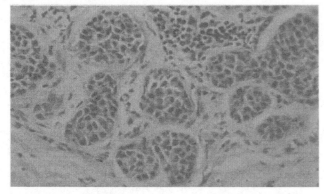

Figure 5.19 Lobular carcinoma *in situ*. The ductules and acini are distended with loosely arranged, spheroidal and angulated cells, and their lumina have been obliterated. The tumour cells have small, pleomorphic, hyperchromatic nuclei and eosinophilic cytoplasm. There is no stromal invasion. Compare with Figures 5.16–5.18.   H & E × 240

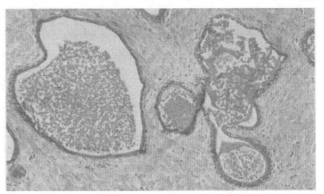

Figure 5.20 Cystic disease of the breast. Section showing irregularly shaped cysts containing eosinophilic, proteinaceous coagulum. There is no epitheliosis.   H & E × 96

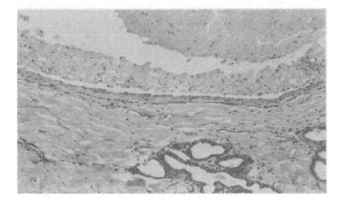

Figure 5.21 Cystic disease of the breast. The lumen of the cyst in the upper half of the field contains foam cells and proteinaceous fluid. The epithelial lining is compressed and markedly attenuated.   H & E × 96

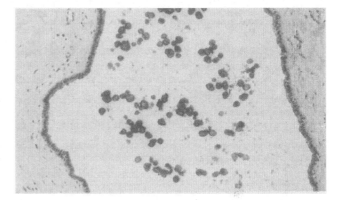

Figure 5.22 Cystic disease with calcification of luminal contents. Part of a cyst showing numerous basophilic, granular deposits of calcium in the lumen.   H & E × 96

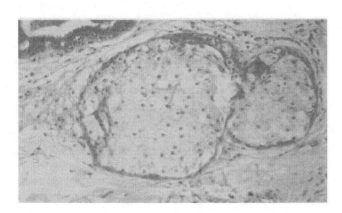

Figure 5.23 Cystic disease of the breast. Section showing a small cyst whose lumen is filled with cells which have voluminous, foamy cytoplasm. H & E × 240

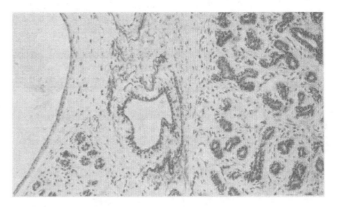

Figure 5.24 Distribution of elastic fibres in mammary lobule, duct and cyst. The photomicrograph shows a lobule, a duct and part of a cyst. Elastic fibres are present in the wall of the duct, but not around the acini and ductules of the lobule nor in the wall of the cyst. This suggests that the cysts of mammary cystic hyperplasia originate from the terminal intralobular ductules rather than from the extralobular ducts.   Orcein elastic stain × 96

above. These cells may also proliferate around the ducts as illustrated in Figure 5.15. In carcinoma *in situ* there is no such myoepithelial hyperplasia, and the cells may be difficult to identify as they become progressively attenuated by being stretched around the distended duct. Periductal changes, in the form of fibrosis and inflammatory cell infiltration, are more usually associated with *in situ* carcinoma, but may be present in benign hyperplasia, particularly if there has been leakage of cyst contents into the surrounding tissue. Again, periductal elastosis is seen more frequently in carcinoma *in situ* but may occur in benign hyperplasia.

Atypical Lobular Hyperplasia

A particular pattern of benign hyperplasia affecting the peripheral acini of the lobules and termed 'atypical lobular hyperplasia' or 'atypical lobule type B' is illustrated in Figures 5.16–5.18. This can be extremely difficult to distinguish from lobular carcinoma *in situ* (Figure 5.19). Although some of the diagnostic criteria of the latter condition are present, the total picture falls short of true lobular carcinoma *in situ* (Figure 5.19). There is usually only partial lobular involvement with less distension of the acini and some persistence of the lumina. The appearance of the proliferating cells within the lumina of the acini is less uniform than the monotonous pattern seen in lobular carcinoma *in situ* and the cells are more crowded, without the lack of cohesion so typical of lobular carcinoma *in situ*. Atypical lobular hyperplasia is frequent in breasts in which fully developed lobular carcinoma *in situ* or infiltrating lobular carcinoma is present elsewhere.

Relationship of Benign Epithelial Hyperplasia to Cancer

In studies correlating benign breast disease with the subsequent risk of cancer development, lesions with epithelial hyperplasia have usually been found to be associated with an increased risk[3–7]. However, in some studies, cystic disease with or without epithelial hyperplasia has also been found to be associated with a higher risk of subsequent carcinoma[8]. In the study of Page *et al.*[5], atypical lobular hyperplasia carried a higher risk than most other forms of benign epithelial hyperplasia occurring in the cystic disease complex. Page and colleagues[5] also found that, as well as the more usual epithelial hyperplasia, apocrine change with papillary tufting was significant. Haagensen[8] also noted that subsequent carcinoma was more frequent in patients with gross cystic disease in which apocrine metaplasia was found at biopsy. Some studies suggest that the risk of cancer is increased in women with epithelial hyperplasia if histological calcification is present in the lesion[6]. However, there is still controversy concerning the relative risk of carcinoma in women with benign breast disease, both with regard to the significance of different histological features of benign breast disease, and indeed as to whether there is any increased risk at all[2].

Cysts

Cysts vary greatly in size from microscopic to macroscopic dimensions. They may be present in combination with epithelial hyperplasia or may be seen alone. The cysts are usually lined by epithelium (Figure 5.20), but this may be lost if the contents are under pressure (Figure 5.21). Metaplastic changes are frequent and many cysts are lined by pink cells; these also may show proliferative changes. Leakage of cyst contents into the surrounding stroma can result in a brisk inflammatory response (see Chapter 3). At low magnification this may be confused initially with infiltrating carcinoma, particularly if the cyst has collapsed and the lumen has been obliterated by the inflammatory cells. Calcification is sometimes seen within the lumen of a cyst (Figure 5.22), and foam cells may also be present (Figure 5.23). Usually elastic tissue cannot be demonstrated in the wall of a cyst, and this is taken by some authorities[1] to indicate that cysts arise from lobules rather than from extralobular ducts (Figure 5.24).

References

1. Azzopardi, J. G. (1979). *Problems in Breast Pathology*, p. 23. (Vol. 11 in Bennington, J. L. (consulting ed.) *Major Problems in Pathology*.) (London, Philadelphia and Toronto: Saunders)

2 Love, S. M., Gelman, R. S. and Silen, W. (1982). Fibrocystic 'disease' of the breast – a non disease? *N. Engl. J. Med.*, **307**, 1010

3. Wellings, S. R., Jensen, H. M. and Marcum, R. G. (1975). An atlas of subgross pathology of the human breast with special reference to possible precancerous lesions *J. Natl. Cancer Inst.*, **55**, 231

4. Black, M. M., Barclay, T. H. C., Cutler, S. J., Hankey, B. F. and Asire, A. J. (1972). Association of atypical characteristics of benign breast lesions with subsequent risk of breast cancer. *Cancer*, **29**, 338

5. Page, D. L., Zwaag, R. V., Rogers, L. W., Williams, L. T., Walker, W. E. and Hartmann, W. H. (1978). Relation between component parts of fibrocystic disease complex and breast cancer. *J. Natl. Cancer Inst.*, **61**, 1055

6. Hutchinson, W. B., Thomas, D. B., Hamlin, W .B., Roth, G. J., Peterson, A. V. and Williams, B. (1980). Risk of breast cancer in women with benign breast disease. *J. Natl. Cancer Inst.*, **65**, 13

7. Jensen, H. M. (1981). Breast pathology, emphasizing precancerous and cancer-associated lesions. In Bulbrook, R. D. and Taylor, D. J. (eds.) *Commentaries on Research in Breast Disease*, Vol. 2, p. 41. (New York: Liss)

8. Haagensen, C. D., Bodian, C. and Haagensen, D. E. Jr. (1981). *Breast Carcinoma. Risk and Detection*, p. 55. (Philadelphia, London and Toronto: Saunders)

Cystic Disease Complex 2

The term 'adenosis' has been used to designate both an increase in the number of lobular ductules or acini and an alteration in the architecture of these structures, as in blunt duct adenosis. Although usually seen in association with cystic hyperplasia the various forms of adenosis may occur alone.

Sclerosing Adenosis

The most widely recognized form of adenosis is sclerosing adenosis. The condition is now well known but in the past was sometimes confused with infiltrating carcinoma. Even with cognizance of the problem, diagnostic difficulties can still arise. The process consists of proliferation of epithelium, myoepithelium and stroma. There is retention of the overall lobular architecture and the lesion has a sharply demarcated edge; both these features can be recognized at low magnification (Figures 6.1 and 6.2). The stroma is usually densely collagenous, often with abundant elastic tissue, disrupts the normal lobular architecture and compresses the acini to produce a pseudomalignant pattern (Figures 6.2–6.5). However, in many of the tubules well-defined double cell layers are apparent, and the presence of abundant myoepithelium can be demonstrated by staining for alkaline phosphatase (Figures 6.6–6.8). Pink cell (apocrine) metaplasia is sometimes prominent (Figure 6.9) and microcalcification may be present (Figures 6.6 and 6.10). In some forms of sclerosing adenosis the epithelial component predominates, producing nodules of proliferating glandular elements (Figure 6.2). Invasion of nerves and vessels have both been described in sclerosing adenosis[1,2]. The former is illustrated in Figure 6.11.

Radial Scar

Another important variant of sclerosing adenosis is illustrated in Figures 6.12–6.16. This is known variously as radial scar, sclero-elastotic scar, stellate scar, or non-encapsulated sclerosing lesion, and is similar, if not identical, to the sclerosing adenosis with pseudo-infiltration, and infiltrating epitheliosis, of other authors[3]. The stroma in these lesions contains abundant elastic tissue (Figure 6.4) and the resulting radial scar resembles a carcinoma both on gross and mammographic examination; the similarity is accentuated by the frequent presence of calcification. The central sclerotic area is surrounded by foci of epithelial hyperplasia, resulting in an appearance which has been likened to a flower with petals around a stalk. The true significance of this lesion is still controversial: although it is considered entirely benign by many authorities,

others consider it to be premalignant and Linell and colleagues[4] claim that most if not all carcinomas arise from these benign sclerotic lesions. In distinguishing sclerosing adenosis and radial scars from carcinoma, particularly tubular carcinoma, the demonstration of myoepithelial mantles and PAS-positive basement membranes around the tubules of a benign lesion are valuable diagnostic criteria, although either may be indistinct or defective around individual tubules (see Figures 6.17 and 6.18). For further discussion of the microscopic differentiation of sclerosing adenosis, including radial scars, from carcinoma, see Chapter 14.

Blunt Duct Adenosis

Another well recognized form of adenosis is blunt duct adenosis[5]. In this condition there is little or no increase in the number of acini but they show marked dilatation, irregularity of outline and hypertrophy of both epithelium and myoepithelium (Figure 6.19). Although epithelial hyperplasia may be present, it is not usually a prominent feature. The inner epithelial cells often show apocrine snouting, sometimes termed 'columnar metaplasia'. There is usually an accompanying increase in the specialized connnective tissue stroma of the lobule. As in other benign lesions, the tubules have double-cell layers, a feature which distinguishes blunt duct adenosis from infiltrating carcinoma.

Microglandular Adenosis

The term 'microglandular adenosis'[5] has been used to describe the rare condition illustrated in Figure 6.20. Proliferating tubules lie within adipose tissue or within a fibrous stroma which is usually rich in collagen, sparsely cellular and often hyalinized. The appearance can easily be mistaken for a well-differentiated (tubular) carcinoma. The clinical and the microscopic features have been described in detail in two recent publications[6,7]. The lesion may be found incidentally on histological examination or may present clinically as a palpable mass. The tubules are usually small, regular and rounded and their lumina contain PAS-positive, diastase-resistant material, occasionally with calcium deposition. The cells lining the tubules are cuboidal or flattened, with clear or eosinophilic cytoplasm which may contain glycogen. Although the presence of a double cell layer is in general an important feature of benign breast lesions, in microglandular adenosis myoepithelial mantles have not been demonstrated. PAS-positive basement membrane material is also usually absent, but the tubules are surrounded by complete reticulin rings as shown by silver impregnation tech-

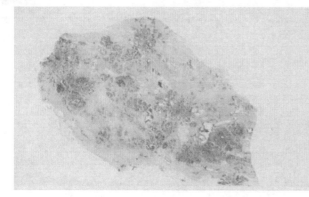

Figure 6.1 Sclerosing adenosis. Section at low magnification showing the lobular distribution of the proliferative process. A radial scar is also present (arrowed). H & E × 2.4

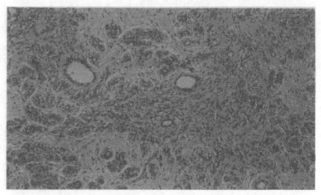

Figure 6.2 Sclerosing adenosis. In this field, proliferation of eosinophilic spindle shaped myoepithelial cells is a prominent feature; the majority of the tubules are compressed and consequently their lumina are inconspicuous. H & E × 96

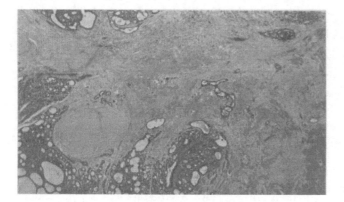

Figure 6.3 Sclerosing adenosis. Section showing part of the central area of a lesion which displays dense fibrosis with hyalinization and prominent elastosis. Distorted lobules are grouped at the periphery. Some tubules are trapped and distorted within the fibrous tissue. H & E × 24

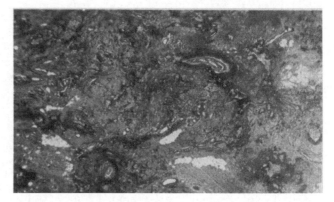

Figure 6.4 Sclerosing adenosis with elastosis. Section showing abundant elastic fibres, distributed both around the ducts and irregularly within the fibrous stroma. Elastin is stained black; collagen is red. Verhoeff's elastic stain/Van Gieson × 96

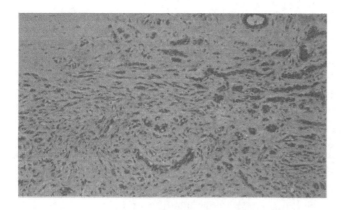

Figure 6.5 Sclerosing adenosis. In this lesion fibrosis has compressed the epithelial component into small tubules and narrow columns of cells, producing a pattern which might suggest infiltrating carcinoma. H & E × 96

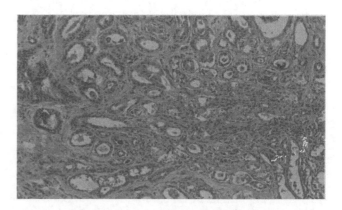

Figure 6.6 Sclerosing adenosis. There is a proliferation of both juxtaluminal and myoepithelial cells. Many of the tubules display distinct double cell layers and show pink cell (apocrine) metaplasia. Small deposits of calcium are present in the lumina of a few tubules. H & E × 96

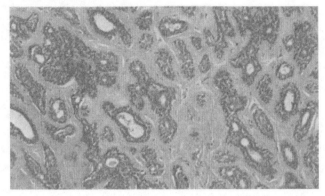

Figure 6.7 Sclerosing adenosis. Proliferation of tubular structures in a dense, hyaline, fibrous stroma. Most of the tubules display very conspicuous double cell layers.   H & E × 96

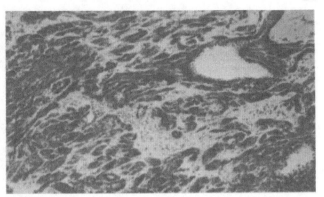

Figure 6.8 Sclerosing adenosis. Myoepithelial cells, stained red, are prominent around the tubules and in places form the most conspicuous component of the lesion. Azo coupling technique for alkaline phosphatase × 96

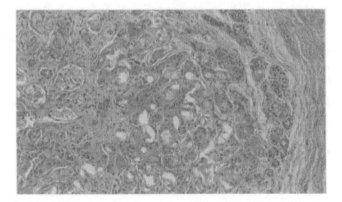

Figure 6.9 Sclerosing adenosis. Part of an altered lobule within a large area of sclerosing adenosis. Here the juxtaluminal cells have undergone marked pink cell metaplasia.   H & E × 96

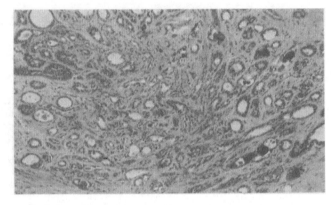

Figure 6.10 Sclerosing adenosis. The combination of epithelial proliferation, myoepithelial proliferation and fibrosis has produced marked distortion of the normal architecture. There are multiple foci of microcalcification, particularly in the right half of the field.   H & E × 96

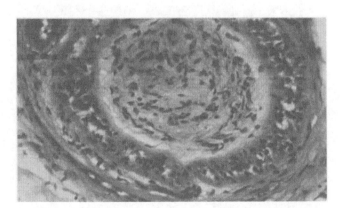

Figure 6.11 Sclerosing adenosis, with perineural extension. The lesion had the typical microscopic features of sclerosing adenosis. In the area shown here an epithelial tubule encircles a small nerve.   H & E × 240

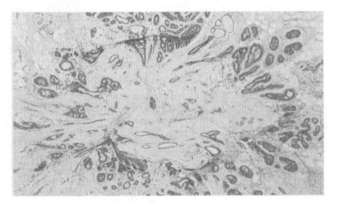

Figure 6.12 Radial scar. Section showing the typical microarchitecture: a central area of sclerosis with entrapment of tubules, and a peripheral corona of ducts some of which display a tendency to radial orientation.   H & E × 24

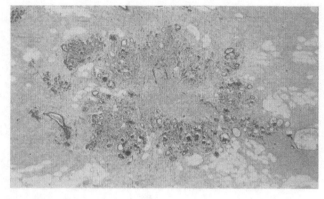

Figure 6.13 Radial scar. This section shows a central area of fibrosis and elastosis, surrounded by a corona of small, irregularly arranged tubules, with intraluminal calcium deposits. H & E × 24

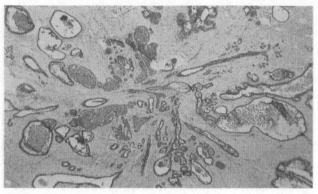

Figure 6.14 Radial scar. The lesion illustrated here is a typical 'radial scar'. Ducts radiate outwards from a central focus, and become dilated peripherally. In some places the lumina are filled with proliferated epithelial cells. H & E × 24

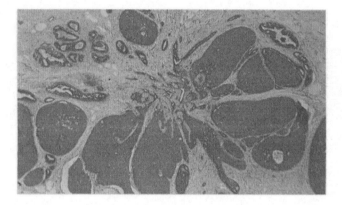

Figure 6.15 Radial scar. Another example of a radial scar showing the typical 'flower-head' pattern. In this lesion, epithelial hyperplasia has resulted in many of the ducts becoming filled with solid masses of cells. H & E × 24

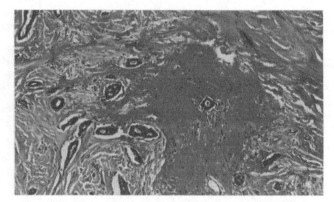

Figure 6.16 Radial scar, with prominent elastosis. Part of a lesion which had the typical general features of a radial scar. In the centre of the lesion there is entrapment of epithelial tubules in a dense fibroelastic stroma. The elastin is stained deeply with eosin. In this field, the appreances may be considered suggestive of a well-differentiated infiltrating tubular carcinoma, but the ducts have retained their double cell layers. H & E × 96

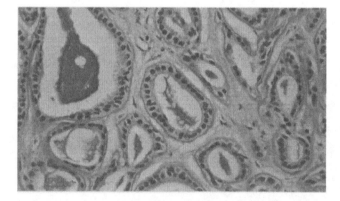

Figure 6.17 Basement membranes around benign ductules. Here the myo-epithelial cells are inconspicuous but, in this section, stained by the PAS technique, all the tubules are surrounded by delicate basement membranes, stained pink. Such basement membranes are absent in tubular carcinoma, so the stain may be helpful in diagnosis. PAS × 240

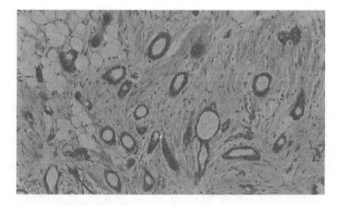

Figure 6.18 Tubular carcinoma. Section of a tumour, 1 cm in diameter, excised from the breast of a 45-year-old woman. The neoplasm is composed of highly-differentiated epithelial tubules, growing in a fibroblastic stroma. In the top left corner of the field, the growth has invaded the mammary adipose tissue. The tumour cells are regular in size, shape and staining properties, and mitotic figures are very infrequent. The high degree of differentiation may suggest a benign lesion, but the neoplastic tubules lack double cell layers and regular basement membranes. H & E × 96

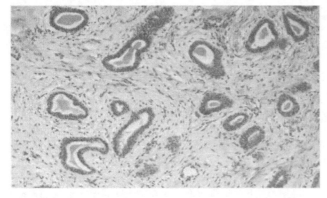

Figure 6.19 Blunt duct adenosis. Section showing proliferation of ducts which end blindly and do not branch out to form lobular structures. There is a moderately cellular fibroblastic stroma. The ducts display double cell layers. H & E × 96

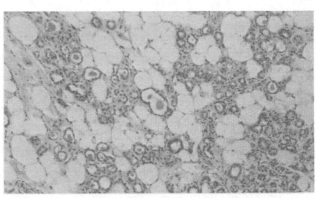

Figure 6.20 Microglandular adenosis. This microscopic lesion was found incidentally in a breast lump which otherwise had the features of conventional cystic hyperplasia. There are irregular clusters of small, fully differentiated tubules, lying amidst adipose tissue. The tubules are, for the most part, lined by a single layer of cuboidal cells. The lumina contain some eosinophilic secretion. There is no fibroblastic stromal response such as occurs in tubular carcinoma. H & E × 96

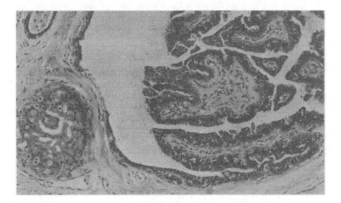

Figure 6.21 Papilloma of peripheral mammary duct. Sections of a papilloma arising in a small peripheral duct. The fronds have thick fibrovascular cores and are covered by double cell layers of epithelium. H & E × 96

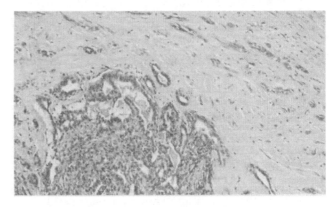

Figure 6.22 Sclerosing peripheral intraduct papilloma. The papilloma in the lower left portion of the field has undergone considerable sclerosis and many small tubules are trapped in dense fibrous tissue, producing a pattern of spurious invasion. The entrapped epithelial structures extend out for some distance from the main lesion. H & E × 24

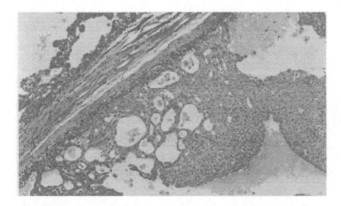

Figure 6.23 Juvenile papillomatosis of the breast. A breast lesion from an 18-year-old girl. The distended duct on the right is partly filled with epithelial cells and many of the cells in the duct on the left display apocrine metaplasia. The cribriform spaces are very irregular in size and shape. H & E × 96

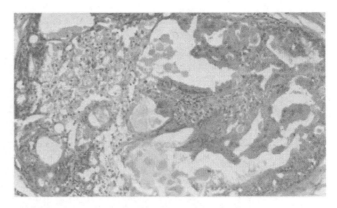

Figure 6.24 Juvenile papillomatosis of the breast. A section of a lesion from a 20-year-old girl. Apocrine metaplasia is prominent and there are irregularly shaped papillary fringes. Other cells have foamy cytoplasm. The lumen of the cyst also contains eosinophilic proteinaceous coagulum. H & E × 96

niques[6]. Differentiation from tubular carcinoma is discussed in Chapter 14.

Peripheral Papilloma

Small benign papillomas in peripheral ducts are also frequently seen as part of the cystic disease complex (Figure 6.21). Sometimes they are composed entirely of apocrine cells but otherwise they do not differ histologically from the larger papillomas seen in more proximal ducts, described in Chapter 9. Sclerosis of such lesions as in larger duct papillomas can produce a picture easily confused with infiltrating carcinoma (Figure 6.22).

Juvenile Papillomatosis

The term 'juvenile papillomatosis' has been applied by Rosen and colleagues[8] to a clinically well-circumscribed lesion characterized histologically by cysts and florid hyperplastic changes, occurring in the mammary ducts and lobules of adolescents and young women. Rosen et al.[9] have now reviewed 84 cases with a mean age of 21 years (range 10–44 years); 69% were 20 years or under. The lesions were usually diagnosed clinically as fibroadenoma. On gross examination the numerous holes, corresponding microscopically to cysts and dilated ducts, result in an appearance which has been likened to Swiss cheese.

Histologically there are cysts with florid hyperplasia and papillomatosis of both apocrine and non-apocrine types (Figures 6.23 and 6.24) sometimes with severe atypia. Areas of sclerosing adenosis and duct stasis with collections of foamy histiocytes are also present. Rare foci of comedo-type necrosis and occasional mitotic figures may be seen. So far there have been no reports of carcinoma developing after excision biopsy of juvenile papillomatosis, but follow-up in many cases has been relatively short. However, Rosen et al.[8] recorded three patients who had concurrent carcinoma and, in their larger review[9], found that 26% of patients for whom information was available had a family history of breast cancer. They recommend long term follow-up of all patients with juvenile papillomatosis.

References

1. Taylor, H. B. and Norris, H. J. (1967). Epithelial invasion of nerves in benign diseases of the breast. *Cancer*, **20**, 2245

2. Eusebi, V. and Azzopardi, J. G. (1976). Vascular infiltration in benign breast disease. *J. Pathol.*, **118**, 9

3. Azzopardi, J. G. (1979). *Problems in Breast Pathology*, p. 174. (Vol. 11 in Bennington, J. L. (consulting ed.) *Major Problems in Pathology*, (London, Philadelphia and Toronto: Saunders)

4. Linell, F., Ljungberg, D. and Andersson, I. (1980). Breast carcinoma: aspects of early stages, progression and related problems. *Acta Pathol. Microbiol. Scand. A., Suppl.* 272

5. McDivitt, R. W., Stewart, F. W. and Berg, J. W. (1968). Tumours of the breast. In *Atlas of Tumour Pathology, 2nd series, Fascicle 2*, p. 91. (Washington DC: Armed Forces Institute of Pathology)

6. Clement, P. B. and Azzopardi, J. G. (1983). Microglandular adenosis of the breast – a lesion simulating tubular carcinoma. *Histopathology*, **7**, 169

7. Rosen, P. P. (1983). Microglandular adenosis. A benign lesion simulating invasive mammary carcinoma. *Am. J. Surg. Pathol.* **7**, 137

8. Rosen, P. P., Cantrell, B., Mullen, D. L. and De Palo, A. (1980). Juvenile papillomatosis (Swiss cheese disease) of the breast. *Am. J. Surg. Pathol.*, **4**, 3

9. Rosen, P. P., Lyngholm, B., Kinne, D. W. and Beattie E. J. Jr. (1982). Juvenile papillomatosis of the breast and family history of breast carcinoma. *Cancer*, **49**, 2591

Fibroadenoma, Variants of Fibroadenoma, Benign Cystosarcoma Phyllodes Tumour, Mammary Adenoma and Adenoma of the Nipple

7

Fibroadenoma

This common benign mammary neoplasm is the most frequent reason for breast biopsy in young women in the third and early fourth decade. However, they are also occasionally seen in older women. Fibroadenomas are usually single but are multiple in about 20% of cases.

Pathological Features

Fibroadenomas are thought to arise from the lobules and are considered by many pathologists to represent an exaggerated form of lobular hyperplasia. On gross examination they present a characteristic appearance, with a well-defined rounded or lobulated outline clearly demarcated from the adjacent tissue, from which the neoplasm protrudes when cut across (Figure 7.1). Microscopically, fibroadenomas are seen to be composed of both fibrous stroma and glandular tissue; the latter displays a double layer comprising epithelium and myoepithelium (Figure 7.2). In the past these neoplasms have been classified according to the arrangement of the stroma relative to the epithelial component: in the pericanalicular variety the stroma surrounds, but does not distort, the epithelial tubules (Figure 7.2), whereas in the intracanalicular type the stroma compresses and appears to grow into the epithelial spaces (Figure 7.3). However, this classification appears to have little clinical significance and many tumours show a mixed pattern.

Fibroadenomas hardly ever give rise to diagnostic difficulties but occasionally the marked variations in pattern which can occur in both epithelial and stromal elements may be confusing.

Variations in Epithelial Component

Apocrine metaplasia of the epithelial component is common (Figure 7.4). Squamous metaplasia is rare. The changes of sclerosing adenosis are seen quite frequently (Figure 7.5). During pregnancy and lactation the epithelium may display secretory changes (Figure 7.6). In Figure 7.7, there is hyperplasia of the epithelial component; this is a relatively common finding and is sometimes quite marked. On the other hand, atrophy of the epithelium is less common but may be seen in fibroadenomas from older women when occasionally the epithelial component disappears from large areas of the neoplasm.

Carcinoma Arising in a Fibroadenoma

Very rarely, carcinoma may arise within a fibroadenoma[1]. The malignant epithelial changes may be confined to the fibroadenoma or involve epithelium both within and around the lesion. Lobular carcinoma *in situ* (Figures 7.8 and 7.9) is more frequent that *in situ* duct carcinoma. This is to be expected if fibroadenomas arise from the lobules. In distinguishing between epithelial hyperplasia and *in situ* carcinoma, the same criteria apply in fibroadenomas as elsewhere in the breast. A fibroadenoma may also be involved secondarily by an infiltrating carcinoma, as shown in Figure 7.10.

Recently four cases of lobular endocrine neoplasia within fibroadenomas have been described by Eusebi and Azzopardi[2]. The tumours were identified by light microscopic, silver impregnation and ultrastructural studies. Argyrophilia and the presence of dense-core granules established the identity of the tumour type. The tumours were *in situ* and the authors considered them distinct from, but very probably related to, lobular carcinoma *in situ*.

Variations in the Stromal Component

Variations in the mesenchymal component also occur. The stroma is usually fibroblastic (Figure 7.2) but varies from a highly myxoid pattern (Figure 7.3) to the densely hyaline appearance shown in Figure 7.11. This latter feature is seen most commonly in fibroadenomas from older women often in association with atrophy of the epithelium, consistent with the view that fibroadenomas eventually regress in older women if left untreated. Calcification of the stroma can occur (Figure 7.12) and osseous and cartilaginous metaplasia have been described; again these changes are usually seen in older patients. The presence of adipose tissue within the stroma may result from the incorporation of pre-existing fat or possibly from metaplasia. Rarely, smooth muscle is present in the stroma of a fibroadenoma. Sarcomatous change in fibroadenomas is discussed in Chapter 21.

Another change which can give rise to diagnostic difficulty is infarction within a fibroadenoma. This is seen most frequently during pregnancy.

Variants of Fibroadenoma

Giant Fibroadenoma

The meaning attached to this term varies: to some it indicates a microscopically typical fibroadenoma which is unusual only because of its large size, while, to others, it is synonymous with a benign cystosarcoma

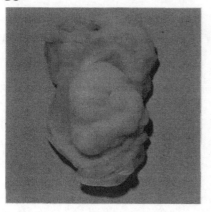

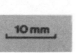

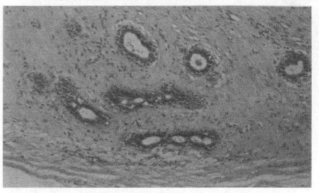

Figure 7.1 Fibroadenoma. A lesion excised from the breast of a 28-year-old woman. The tumour is sharply defined, has a lobulated appearance and bulges from the surrounding mammary tissue

Figure 7.2 Fibroadenoma. In this field the growth pattern is of the pericanalicular type. Part of the capsule is seen at the bottom of the photograph. A double cell layer is apparent in some tubules.   H & E × 96

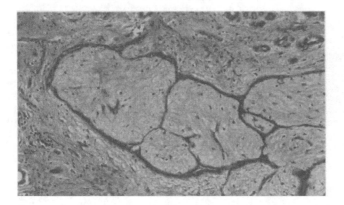

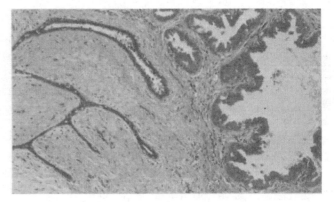

Figure 7.3 Fibroadenoma. Section showing a typical intracanalicular arrangement. The epithelial tubules form a complex branching pattern with apparent encirclement of stromal nodules. In this lesion the stroma is myxoid, being sparsely cellular but rich in basophilic connective tissue mucin. H & E × 96

Figure 7.4 Fibroadenoma with pink cell metaplasia. A tumour in which the epithelial component has undergone pink cell (apocrine) metaplasia. A conventional intracanalicular pattern is present on the left: on the right the tubules are dilated and display prominent pink cell change.   H & E × 96

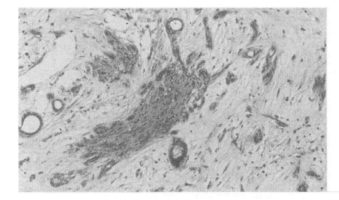

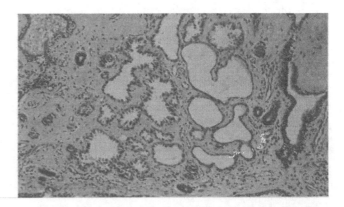

Figure 7.5 Fibroadenoma with focal sclerosing adenosis. Part of a mammary nodule which elsewhere had the microscopic features of a conventional fibroadenoma with mixed pericanalicular and intracanalicular pattern. In this field, myoepithelial proliferation is very prominent, the cells having brightly eosinophilic cytoplasm.   H & E × 96

Figure 7.6 Fibroadenoma with focal lactational change. The ductules in the centre of the field are dilated and their epithelium exhibits secretory activity. Other ducts, such as those on the right and left, have not responded. H & E × 96

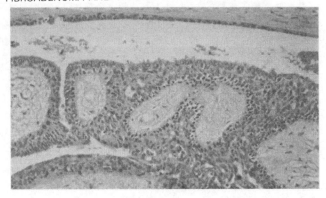

Figure 7.7 Fibroadenoma with epithelial proliferation. Part of an intracanalicular fibroadenoma in which epithelial proliferation is unusually pronounced. The changes do not correspond with any recognized pattern of *in situ* carcinoma, and are considered to represent epitheliosis affecting fibroadenomatous epithelium. H & E × 96

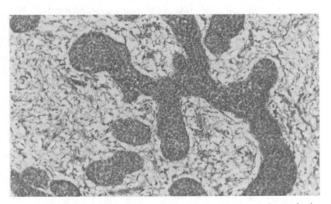

Figure 7.8 Fibroadenoma with the development of lobular carcinoma *in situ*. An area of the tumour showing the characteristic features of an intracanalicular fibroadenoma with a loose myxoid stroma. H & E × 96

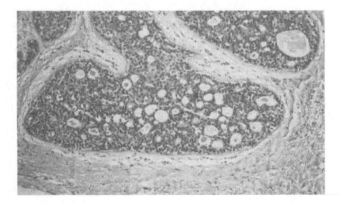

Figure 7.9 Fibroadenoma with the development of *in situ* carcinoma. Macroscopically this tumour was a typical encapsulated fibroadenoma. The microscopic structure was predominantly that of an intracanalicular growth pattern without undue epithelial proliferation. However some areas, as illustrated here, showed distension of the ductules with masses of carcinoma cells featuring a cribriform pattern. Although such a pattern is more typical of intraduct carcinoma, the cytological features in this lesion are more suggestive of lobular carcinoma. H & E × 96

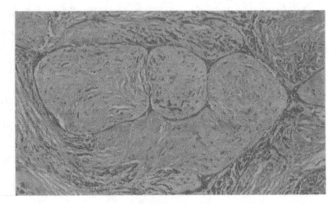

Figure 7.10 Fibroadenoma invaded by lobular carcinoma. Section of a fribroadenoma invaded by lobular carcinoma which has arisen in the surrounding breast. The section shows part of an intracanalicular fibroadenoma with infiltrating columns of small, darkly-staining, lobular carcinoma cells. H & E × 96

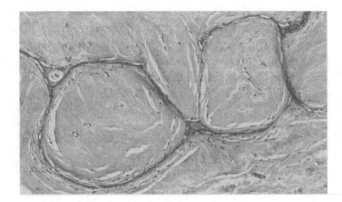

Figure 7.11 Fibroadenoma. In this tumour the stroma is sparsely cellular, with abundant hyalinized collagen. The growth pattern is intracanalicular. H & E × 96

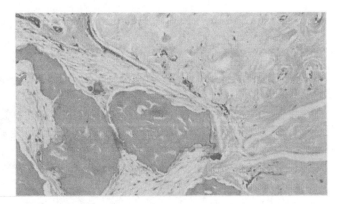

Figure 7.12 Fibroadenoma. Here the epithelial component has undergone marked atrophy. The stroma is sparsely cellular and displays prominent hyalinization with focal calcification. H & E × 96

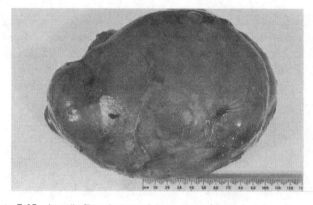

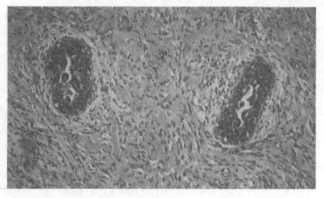

Figure 7.13 Juvenile fibroadenoma. A large encapsulated mass from the breast of a 9-year-old girl

Figure 7.14 Juvenile fibroadenoma. Section of the tumour illustrated in Figure 7.13. The growth pattern is pericanalicular and the epithelium shows some proliferation with piling up of the cells. The stroma is moderately cellular, it is loose immediately around the tubules, but is denser, with abundant collagen, between the tubules.   H & E × 96

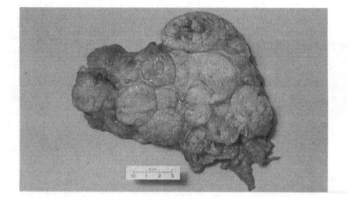

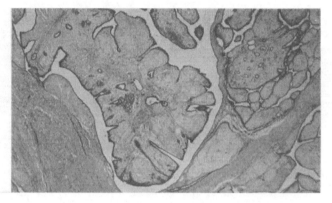

Figure 7.15 Benign (cystosarcoma) phyllodes tumour. A large tumour from the breast of a 52-year-old woman. The photograph shows the cut surface of the neoplasm, featuring prominent gross lobulation, a glistening mucoid appearance and micronodulation as a result of clefting along the epithelial spaces

Figure 7.16 Benign (cystosarcoma) phyllodes tumour. Section of a large mass excised from the breast of a 55-year-old woman. The tumour has a very prominent intracanalicular pattern, with clefting along the epithelial spaces. The stroma is abundant, basophilic and myxoid.   H & E × 24

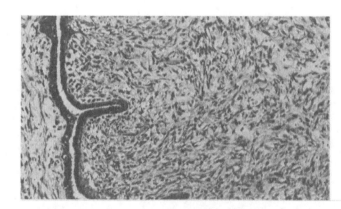

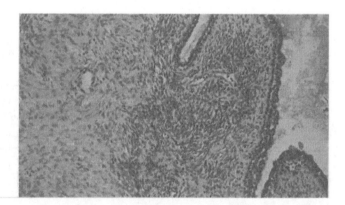

Figure 7.17 Benign (cystosarcoma) phyllodes tumour. Section of 3 cm-diameter tumour from a 39-year-old woman, showing the characteristic hypercellular stroma and part of a compressed and distorted epithelial component on the left. Although very cellular, the stromal pattern is not that of a sarcoma; nuclear aberration is inconspicuous and mitotic figures are very infrequent.   H & E × 96

Figure 7.18 Benign (cystosarcoma) phyllodes tumour. On the right, there is part of an epithelial tubule showing a distinct double cell layer. The stroma is hypercellular, this feature being especially prominent in a zone adjacent to the epithelium, but the mesenchymal cells are quite regular in size, shape and staining properties, and only a very few mitotic figures could be found. H & E × 96

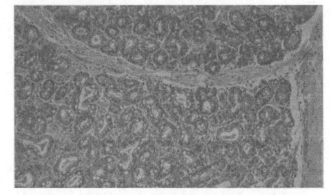

Figure 7.19 Mammary adenoma. Sections of an encapsulated nodule, 1 cm in diameter, from the breast of a 35-year-old woman. The tumour is composed of small rounded acini or tubules, supported by a relatively scanty stroma. At higher magnification, the acini could be seen to have a double cell layer. H & E × 96

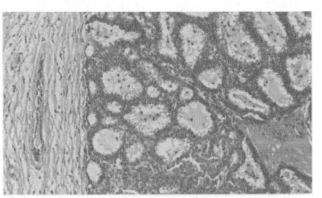

Figure 7.20 Lactating adenoma. Part of a sharply circumscribed nodule excised from the breast of a lactating woman. A thick fibrous capsule is seen on the left. The stroma is very scanty, compared with that of a fibro-adenoma, and the acini display secretory activity with dilatation of the lumina. H & E × 96

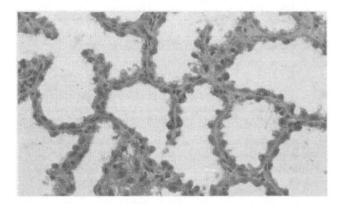

Figure 7.21 Lactating adenoma. This photograph shows more advanced lactational change than those illustrated in Figure 7.20. The acini are markedly distended and the lining cells have assumed a 'hobnail' configuration. Myoepithelial cells are difficult to identify in haematoxylin and eosin preparations, but in sections stained for alkaline phosphatase regular myoepithelial mantles can be readily demonstrated. H & E × 240

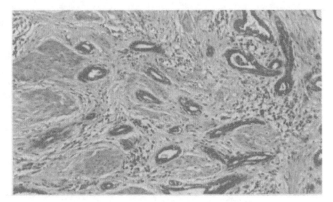

Figure 7.22 Adenoma of the nipple (florid papillomatosis) in a male. Section of a nodule excised from the nipple of a 45-year-old man. Proliferated ducts mingle with smooth muscle bundles, producing a pattern of spurious invasive growth. Many of the tubules feature double cell layers, indicating the benign nature of the lesion. H & E × 96

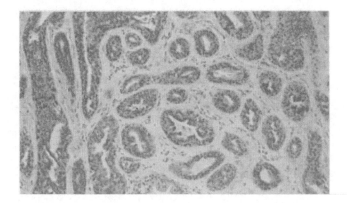

Figure 7.23 Adenoma of the nipple. In this lesion tubule formation is prominent and double cell layers are clearly seen. H & E × 96

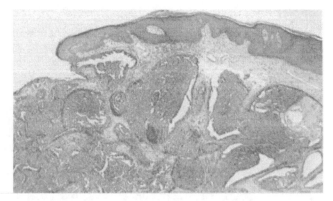

Figure 7.24 Adenoma of the nipple. A photomicrograph at low magnification, showing the epidermis of the nipple at the top, and the subjacent adenoma comprising proliferating duct epithelium displaying solid and papillary growth patterns with irregularly shaped lumina. H & E × 24

phyllodes tumour. The large fibroadenomas seen in adolescents – the so-called juvenile fibroadenomas – have also been called giant fibroadenomas.

Juvenile Fibroadenoma

Fibroadenomas in adolescents are usually similar to those seen in adults, but some grow rapidly, reach a large size and produce marked distortion of the breast. There is often dilatation of superficial veins, and the overlying skin may be stretched and thin. The macroscopic appearance of a typical example is illustrated in Figure 7.13. Histologically the appearances are variable. A predominantly pericanalicular pattern may be present, often with hyperplastic epithelium and a stroma which is more cellular than that of fibroadenomas in adults (Figure 7.14). However, the degree of stromal cellularity does not reach that of cystosarcoma phyllodes tumours, from which juvenile fibroadenomas should be distinguished. Sometimes the microscopic appearances are simply those of prominent lobular hyperplasia. On other occasions the lesions show similar changes to those seen in virginal hypertrophy. Indeed it has been suggested that some juvenile fibroadenomas represent localized areas of virginal hypertrophy[3]. Juvenile fibroadenomas are usually single, and recurrence after excision is rare; but rapid recurrence following excision has been described in a group of patients with multiple, and often bilateral, tumours[3].

Cystosarcoma Phyllodes (Phyllodes Tumour)

The term 'cystosarcoma phyllodes' has caused considerable confusion since it was originally introduced by Muller in 1838[4] to describe a large fleshy tumour with a papillary leaf-like appearance on the cut surface (Figure 7.15). The use of the term 'sarcoma' at that time indicated a 'fleshy' tumour but not necessarily a malignant one. Since the original description by Muller[4], numerous different names have been applied to this type of neoplasm. As the majority of cystosarcoma phyllodes tumours are benign, attempts have been made to apply terms in which the word 'sarcoma' does not feature. The WHO classification adopts the term 'phyllodes tumour'. As a result of the many different names and the variation in histological types of fibroepithelial neoplasms included under these headings by different authors, there is considerable disagreement in the literature regarding the incidence and behaviour of such neoplasms. The term 'cytosarcoma phyllodes' and its synonyms have been used by some authorities to describe any large tumour with the basic architecture of a fibroadenoma. However, the term should be restricted to fibroepithelial neoplasms with the special pattern illustrated in Figures 7.16–7.18. Such tumours do have the basic architecture of a fibroadenoma but the diagnostic feature is the abundant hypercellular stroma. There is usually an exaggerated intracanalicular pattern which is responsible for the papillary appearance of the cut surface. These neoplasms vary in size and, although generally large (over 5 cm), size should not be taken into account in making the diagnosis. Occasionally small lesions have the typical histological appearances described above and large fibroepithelial neoplasms may have the appearance of a conventional fibroadenoma without the hypercellular stroma. Differentiation between conventional fibro-

adenoma and phyllodes tumour is important, as approximately 20% of phyllodes tumours are malignant and even the benign forms tend to recur if inadequately excised.

Pathological Features

On macroscopic examination phyllodes tumours are well-circumscribed, grey to white, firm tumours, with clefting on the cut surface and often areas of myxoid change and necrosis (Figure 7.15). Small protrusions from the external surface are sometimes discernible and when such a neoplasm is enucleated these may be cut through and left behind to give rise to local recurrence. As in conventional fibroadenomas, histological changes may occur in the epithelial or stromal components. Epithelial hyperplasia is moderately frequent and squamous metaplasia is more common than in conventional fibroadenomas. However, apocrine metaplasia is rare and the changes of sclerosing adenosis have not been described in the phyllodes tumour. Variations in the stroma include areas of adipose tissue as well as oedema, myxoid and hyaline change. Calcification and even ossification may also occur. Occasionally areas of conventional fibroadenoma are found within or adjacent to a typical phyllodes tumour. Some authorities consider this to indicate that phyllodes tumours arise from conventional fibroadenomas.

Although most phyllodes tumours are benign, in some the stromal component is malignant. If the strict histological criteria are adhered to, the term 'cystosarcoma phyllodes tumour' is acceptable, but the qualifying terms 'benign' or 'malignant' should always be used. Further discussion of these lesions and differentiation between benign and malignant cystosarcoma phyllodes tumours is given in Chapter 23.

Fibroadenomatoid Hyperplasia

The terms 'fibroadenomatoid hyperplasia' or 'fibroadenomatous hyperplasia' have been used to describe lesions which show the general architecture of a fibroadenoma, but with no clear demarcation from the surrounding breast. Very often, there is cystic disease in the adjacent tissue.

Adenoma of the Breast

Pure mammary adenoma (tubular adenoma), like fibroadenoma, usually occurs in young women. On gross examination the lesion consists of a well-demarcated round nodule with a tan or yellow colour, which is softer than a typical fibroadenoma. Microscopically, a pure adenoma is composed of uniform, closely-packed tubules comprising abundant epithelial cells with surrounding myoepithelial layers (Figure 7.19). Occasional mitotic figures may be present, but there is no cellular atypia. PAS-positive material may be demonstrated within the tubular lumina. The sparse fibrovascular stroma surrounding the tubules sometimes contains lymphocytes. Although there could be difficulty in distinguishing an adenoma from a well-differentiated carcinoma, the presence of a regular myoepithelial layer around the tubules should confirm the diagnosis of adenoma. The suggestion that these lesions are related to the use of oral contraceptives has not been substantiated[5]. A variant, the lactating adenoma, is shown in Figures 7.20 and 7.21. These lesions are similar to tubular adenoma, but occur in pregnant or lactating women, and the tubules are dilated and show secretory activity resulting in alveolar-like patterns. Small foci of necrosis are often present. Hertel *et al.*[5] have described another variant, the combined tubular adenoma and fibroadenoma; these lesions comprise a typical adenoma adjacent to but not intermingling with a conventional fibroadenoma.

Adenoma of the Nipple (Erosive Adenomatosis of Nipple, Florid Papillomatosis of Nipple, Subareolar Duct Papillomatosis, Papillary Adenoma of Nipple)

This relatively uncommon benign tumour is usually unilateral and is most often seen in women in the fourth decade of life. It can also occur in men. Clinically, adenoma of the nipple presents with a discharge, often associated with eczema[6,7]. Other manifestations include swelling or induration of the nipple. Clinical differentiation from Paget's disease may be difficult. Other differential diagnoses include fistula and duct papilloma. Microscopically, adenoma of the nipple consists of duct-like structures supported by connective tissue stroma, occupying the nipple and subareolar areas (Figure 7.22). At low magnification, differentiation from a carcinoma may be difficult, but at high power the two distinct cell layers lining the tubules are easily seen (Figure 7.23). Papillary proliferation and occasional solid areas may be present (Figure 7.24) and sometimes mitotic figures are numerous. Squamous metaplasia, or more rarely apocrine metaplasia, have been described within the lesion. Treatment is by local excision, and although there are rare reports of malignant change affecting a nipple adenoma, the great majority are entirely benign and recurrence is very rare[6,7].

References

1. Fondo, E. Y., Rosen, P. P., Fracchia, A. A. and Urban, J. A. (1979). The problem of carcinoma developing in a fibroadenoma. *Cancer*, **43**, 563

2. Eusebi, V. and Azzopardi, J. G. (1980). Lobular endocrine neoplasia in fibroadenoma of breast. *Histopathology*, **4**, 413

3. Oberman, H. A. (1979). Breast lesions in the adolescent female. In Sommers, S. C. and Rosen, P. P. (eds.) *Pathology Annual*, Vol. 14, Part 1, p. 175. (New York: Appleton-Century-Crofts)

4. Muller, J. (1938). *Uber den feinern Bau und die Formen der krankhaften Geschwulste*, p. 54. (Berlin: G. Reimer)

5. Hertel, B. F., Zaloudek, C. and Kempson, R. L. (1976). Breast adenomas. *Cancer*, **37**, 2891

6. Handley, R. S. and Thackray, A. C. (1962). Adenoma of nipple. *Br. J. Cancer*, **16**, 187

7. Perzin, K. H. and Lattes, R. (1972). Papillary adenoma of the nipple (florid papillomatosis, adenoma, adenomatosis). A clinicopathologic study. *Cancer*, **29**, 996

Miscellaneous Benign Lesions of the Breast   8

Juvenile or Virginal Hypertrophy

Juvenile hypertrophy is an uncommon but distressing condition which can result in rapidly developing, tender, massive breast enlargement in adolescents. It usually involves both breasts, but is occasionally unilateral. The aetiology is obscure as no abnormal hormone levels have been demonstrated in these patients, over half of whom are prepubertal[1]. On histological examination abundant connective tissue is seen surrounding mammary ducts (Figure 8.1). There is usually little or no evidence of lobule formation and the overall appearance is similar to that of gynaecomastia. The stroma, although generally loose and cellular, is sometimes dense and hyalinized. There may be areas of epithelial hyperplasia within the ducts.

Gynaecomastia

The commonest lesion of the male breast is gynaecomastia. It has been reported in association with many different diseases, both endocrine and non-endocrine, and is considered by some to be due to disturbance of the androgen/oestrogen ratio[2]. There is a higher incidence amongst the pubertal and climacteric age groups. There may be diffuse involvement of one or both breasts but gross asymmetry is common, resulting in single or multiple nodules. In the series reported by Bannayan and Hajdu[3] pubertal and hormonal induced lesions tended to be bilateral and diffuse, whereas idiopathic and non-hormonal drug induced lesions were more often unilateral and discrete[2]. The histological changes correlate better with the duration of the condition than with its aetiology. The normal male breast resembles that of a prepubertal female, consisting of a fibro-fatty stroma with ducts but no lobules (Figure 8.2). In its early stages, gynaecomastia displays an increased number of ducts with marked intraductal epithelial proliferation and a cellular vascular, oedematous periductal stroma which may contain lymphocytes and plasma cells (Figures 8.3 and 8.4). When the disease is of long duration the stroma becomes progressively more fibrous and hyaline and regressive changes occur in the epithelium (Figure 8.5). Intermediate phases are also encountered. The hyperplasia of the duct epithelium can be prominent with papillary projections (Figure 8.3) which sometimes may be confused with *in situ* duct carcinoma. However, when *in situ* carcinoma does occur in the male breast it is entirely similar to that seen in the female (Figure 8.6). Lobule formation is unusual in gynaecomastia but does occasionally occur, apparently in the absence of any obvious aetiological factors[3].

Mammary Infarction

Infarction of mammary tissue is not common but is sometimes seen in the hyperplastic breast lobules of pregnant or lactating women. Fibroadenomas may also undergo infarction and again this usually occurs during pregnancy or lactation[4]. Clinically, some of the lesions may be mistaken for a carcinoma. On histological examination the area of ischaemic breast is sharply demarcated from the surrounding tissue with an intervening zone of hyperaemia (Figures 8.7–8.9). Organizing thrombi in veins or arteries may be present. Apart from cases in pregnancy and lactation, there are occasional reports of infarction in non-lactating breasts and haemorrhagic necrosis of the breast has been described in patients receiving anticoagulant therapy[4].

Mammary Lesions due to Primary Vascular Disease

Arteritis is usually a systemic disease which rarely involves the breast, but a few cases have been recorded in which the lesions were predominantly within the breast[5]. The resulting area of induration may be confused on clinical examination with carcinoma. Breast involvement in Wegener's granulomatosis has also been reported[6].

Another vascular lesion which may occasionally simulate mammary carcinoma is thrombophlebitis of the superficial veins of the anterior trunk – Mondor's disease[7].

Hamartoma of the Breast

This relatively uncommon benign mammary lesion has received recent attention because of its very distinctive appearance on mammography as a sharply delineated density[8]. Some of the lesions are impalpable, but clinically they are usually diagnosed as a fibroadenoma. Occasionally, very large lesions can result in marked asymmetry of the breasts (Figure 8.10). The age of patients with this lesion ranges from 15 to 88 years. However, in a large number of cases the condition is first noted during pregnancy or lactation. On gross examination the lesion appears as a well-circumscribed, pseudo-encapsulated, ovoid or disc-like mass of relatively soft breast tissue, and is usually only recognized by the pathologist if the lesion is removed intact (Figure 8.11). Microscopically, it comprises ducts and lobules within a variable stroma consisting of fibrous tissue, occasionally containing smooth muscle and often rich in capillary vessels, interspersed with adipose tissue (Figures 8.12 and 8.13). The glandular elements may show the changes of cystic hyperplasia. The lesion is not a true hamartoma in the sense of a

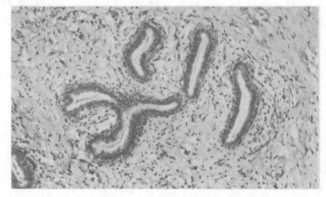

Figure 8.1 Juvenile (virginal) hypertrophy of the breast. A breast biopsy from a 19-year-old girl who had very prominent bilateral mammary enlargement. The section shows a group of irregularly shaped ducts surrounded by loose fibrous connective tissue. There is no formation of acini or lobules. The appearances resemble those seen in gynaecomastia.   H & E × 96

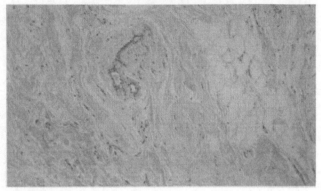

Figure 8.2 Normal male breast. The parenchyma comprises sparse scattered ducts and a fibro-fatty stroma. No lobules are present.   H & E × 96

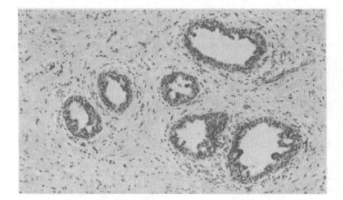

Figure 8.3 Gynaecomastia. Section of an enlarged breast from a 34-year-old man who had bilateral gynaecomastia associated with an interstitial-cell tumour of the testis. There is a cluster of ducts, displaying double cell layers and some proliferation of the juxtaluminal cells with small intraluminal projections. The stroma around the ducts is moderately loose and cellular. H & E × 96

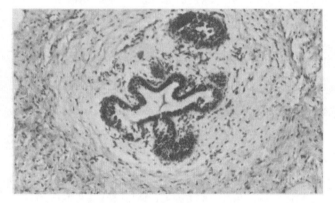

Figure 8.4 Gynaecomastia. Another part of the lesion illustrated in Figure 8.3. The periductal connective tissue is loose and palely staining, in contrast to the denser fibrous tissue further out.   H & E × 96

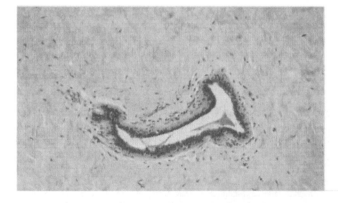

Figure 8.5 Gynaecomastia. Section of an enlarged breast from a 64-year-old man with unilateral gynaecomastia. The duct has a distinct myoepithelial mantle. In contrast to Figures 8.3 and 8.4, there is no epithelial hyperplasia and the surrounding stroma is uniformly dense, with mature collagen. H & E × 96

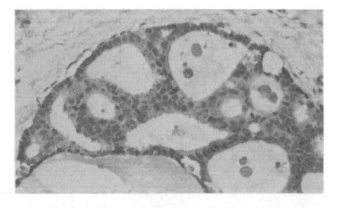

Figure 8.6 Intraduct carcinoma of male breast. A lesion from a 58-year-old man. The section shows a typical cribriform intraduct carcinoma, histologically identical to that commonly seen in the female breast.   H & E × 240

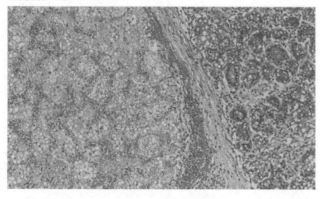

Figure 8.7 Mammary infarction in pregnancy. Sections of a lump excised from the breast of a woman who was in the third trimester of pregnancy. Macroscopically the lesion was well-circumscribed, firm and opaque yellow. The lobule on the right is viable and displays secretory changes associated with late pregnancy. In the left half of the field the epithelial cells have undergone necrosis, but the meshwork of congested blood vessels is still apparent. H & E × 96

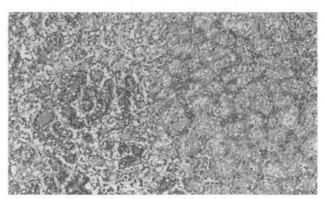

Figure 8.8 Infarction of lactating breast. Section of a lump excised from the breast of a lactating woman. In the right half of the field necrosis is complete, cell outlines are lost and nuclei are reduced to a few pyknotic remnants although erythrocytes are still evident within the capillary network. In the left half of the photomicrograph necrotic changes are less advanced, and there are a few surviving acini containing eosinophilic secretions. H & E × 96

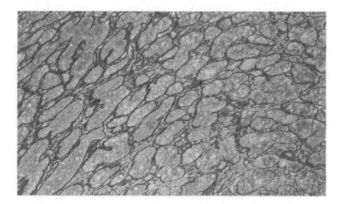

Figure 8.9 Mammary infarction in lactating breast. Macroscopically and microscopically in the haematoxylin and eosin stained sections, the lesion was similar to that illustrated in the previous photomicrograph. This preparation has been stained for reticulin to show the preservation of the connnective tissue framework of the lobule in the infarcted area. Silver impregnation for reticulin × 96

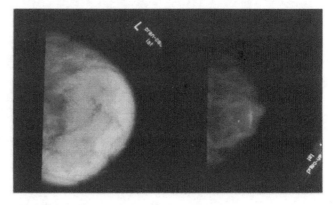

Figure 8.10 Hamartoma of the breast. Bilateral mammograms of a 25-year-old woman with massive distortion of the left breast due to the presence of a large multilobulated mass measuring 15 cm in diameter. The lesion was first noticed during lactation 10 months previously. At operation the relatively soft tumour was easily enucleated from the surrounding breast tissue

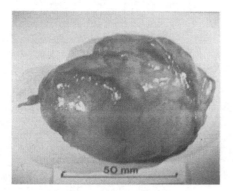

Figure 8.11 Hamartoma of the breast. A pseudo-encapsulated ovoid mass, removed from the breast of a 27-year-old woman, diagnosed clinically as a fibroadenoma. On macroscopic examination the lesion felt softer than a typical fibroadenoma

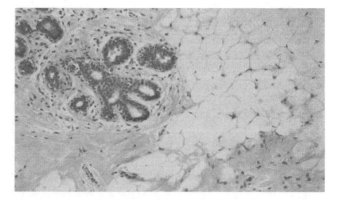

Figure 8.12 Hamartoma of the breast. Section of the mass shown in the previous illustration. Microscopically the lesion consists of a blend of mammary epithelium with both luminal and myoepithelial cells, connective tissue stroma and adipose tissue. Smooth muscle is present in some cases. As seen in the photomicrograph, the histological appearances alone are insufficient to establish the diagnosis of hamartoma, which must depend on a combination of macroscopic features (a sharply-circumscribed mass) and the microscopic findings. The mammographic appearances are also characteristic. H & E × 96

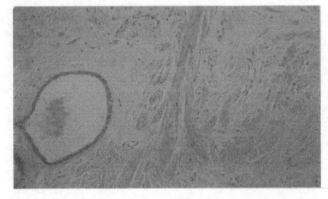

Figure 8.13 Hamartoma of the breast: Sections of another example of mammary hamartoma showing a small cyst and abundant smooth muscle in the stroma.   H & E × 96

Figure 8.14 Fibrosis of the breast. This photomicrograph shows the typical histological features: abundant fibrous tissue with mature collagen and widely scattered fibrocytes. No lobules were present in the affected area, but a single residual duct is seen at the top right hand corner of the field.   H & E × 96

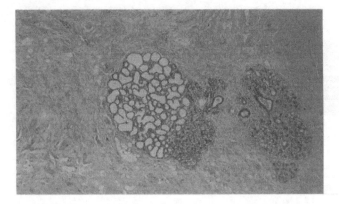

Figure 8.15 Focal pregnancy-like changes. Sections of a breast lesion from a woman who had no history of recent pregnancy or lactation. The lobule to the right of the field is unremarkable: the one in the centre is partly affected by pregnancy-like changes, with marked dilatation of many acini.   H & E × 24

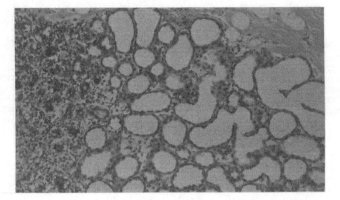

Figure 8.16 Focal pregnancy-like changes. Higher magnification of the affected acini shown in the previous photomicrograph. The dilated secretory acini contrast with the normal acini on the left.   H & E × 96

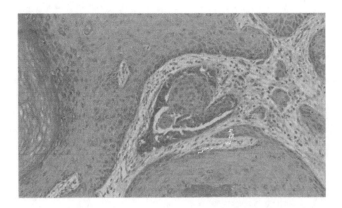

Figure 8.17 Benign squamous metaplasia of mammary ducts. Section of a lesion from the breast of a 22-year-old woman. As illustrated here, some of the ductal epithelium has undergone metaplasia to highly differentiated, stratified squamous epithelium with well-formed stratum granulosum and stratum corneum.   H & E × 96

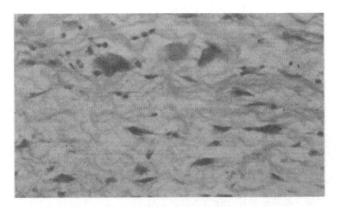

Figure 8.18 Bizarre stromal cells in a benign breast lesion. Section from a biopsy which showed sclerosing adenosis in some areas. Also present were these bizarre, pleomorphic, hyperchromatic and multinucleated stromal cells which do not denote malignancy.   H & E × 240

tumour-like malformation, but appears to be simply an unusually well-circumscribed mass of breast tissue.

Fibrosis of the Breast

This condition has also been called 'chronic indurative mastopathy' or 'chronic indurative mastitis'. The term 'mastitis', implying an inflammatory process, is clearly inappropriate in this context. The conditon usually affects middle-aged women, presenting as an ill-defined mass, most often situated in the upper outer quadrant of the breast. It is characterized by a diffuse increase of sparsely-cellular fibrous tissue, with abundant mature collagen which may show hyalinization. The mammary parenchyma atrophies and becomes very scanty within the lesion (Figure 8.14). Whether this represents a true pathological entity or merely a pattern in the normal involution of the breast is uncertain.

Focal Pregnancy-like Changes

Focal pregnancy-like changes, also known as residual lactating lobules, are a not uncommon incidental finding in breast biopsies from women of all ages. Usually, a single lobule or part of a lobule is involved, the epithelial changes being indistinguishable from those seen in pregnancy and lactation. (Figures 8.15 and 8.16). The only importance of such lesions is that the pleomorphism of the affected cells may occasionally be confused with malignancy, particularly in poorly preserved tissue. There appears to be no definite relationship between either previous pregnancies or hormone therapy: such lesions have been seen many years after the last pregnancy, as well as in nulliparous females and in women who have never received hormone therapy[9].

Squamous Metaplasia

Squamous metaplasia in benign breast disease is rare. It has been reported in fibroadenomas (including phyllodes tumours), duct papillomas and occasionally within otherwise normal ducts or lobules (Figure 8.17).

Benign Stromal Giant Cells

Benign multinucleate stromal giant cells, as shown in Figure 8.18, should not be confused with infiltrating carcinoma. They are usually an incidental finding in biopsies performed for various mammary lesions[10]. Although these cells have been observed in breast specimens from patients with known carcinoma, there is no evidence to suggest that the association is other than coincidental. Their significance is not known.

Amyloid

Rare cases of amyloid pseudotumour confined to the breast have been reported, and amyloid in the breast has also been recorded secondary to rheumatoid arthritis[11,12].

References

1. Oberman, H. A. (1979). Breast lesions in the adolescent female. In Sommers, S. C. and Rosen, P. P. (eds.) *Pathology Annual*, (Vol. 14, Part 1, p. 175. (New York: Appleton-Century-Crofts)

2. Carlson, H. E. (1980). Gynecomastia. *N. Engl. J. Med.*, **303**, 795

3. Bannayan, G. A. and Hajdu, S. I. (1972). Gynecomastia: Clinicopathologic study of 351 cases. *Am. J. Clin. Pathol.*, **57**, 431

4. Azzopardi, J. G. (1979). *Problems in Breast Pathology*, pp. 43, 401. (Vol. 11 in Bennington, J. L. (consulting ed.) *Major Problems in Pathology*.) (London, Philadelphia and Toronto: Saunders)

5. Dega, F. J. and Hunder, G. G. (1974). Vasculitis of the breast. An unusual manifestation of polyarteritis. *Arthr. Rheum.*, **17**, 973

6. Pambakian, H. and Tighe, J. R. (1971). Breast involvement in Wegener's granulomatosis. *J. Clin. Pathol.*, **24**, 343

7. Herrmann, J. R. (1966). Thrombophlebitis of breast and contiguous thoracicoabdominal wall (Mondor's Disease). *NY State J. Med.*, **66**, 3146

8. Linell, F., Ostberg, G., Soderstrom, J., Andersson, I., Hildell, J. and Ljungqvist, U. (1979). Breast hamartomas. An important entity in mammary pathology. *Virchows Arch. A. Pathol. Anat. Hist.*, **383**, 253

9. Kiaer, H. W. and Andersen, J. A. (1977). Focal pregnancy-like changes in the breast. *Acta Pathol. Microbiol. Scand. A*, **85**, 931

10. Rosen, P. P. (1979). Multinucleated mammary stromal giant cells. A benign lesion that simulates invasive carcinoma. *Cancer*. **44**, 1305

11. Fernandez, B. B. and Hernandez, F. J. (1973). Amyloid tumour of the breast. *Arch. Pathol.*, **95**, 102

12. Sadeghee, S. A. and Moore, S. W. (1974). Rheumatoid arthritis, bilaterial amyloid tumours of the breast and multiple cutaneous amyloid nodules. *Am. J. Clin. Pathol.*, **62**, 472

Papillary Lesions of the Breast (Benign and Malignant)

Although the distinction between benign and malignant papillary lesions of the breast usually presents no problem, occasionally it can be extremely difficult. These tumours are, therefore, considered in the same chapter so that their features can be compared and contrasted.

Benign Intraduct Papilloma

Benign papillomas occur most frequently in the large ducts beneath the nipple, where they are usually of sufficient size to be seen macroscopically, but rarely exceed 3 cm in maximum dimension[1]. Occasionally papillomas are seen in the periphery of the duct system, where they tend to be smaller, are often microscopic and may be composed entirely of apocrine-type ('pink') cells. These small peripheral papillomas are usually associated with cystic hyperplasia. Papillomas of the larger ducts frequently present with a nipple discharge, often bloodstained; a mass may or may not be present. On histological examination a benign papilloma has a well-formed branching core of vascular fibrous tissue, covered by a double layer of epithelial cells (Figure 9.1). The outer layer is composed of cuboidal or columnar cells and the inner layer is myoepithelial. The cells adjacent to the lumen may show pink cell metaplasia (Figure 9.2) or more rarely squamous metaplasia. Proliferation of the juxtaluminal or myoepithelial cells can also occur (Figure 9.3). As shown in Figures 9.1 and 9.2, the myoepithelial layer is usually quite evident; although it is sometimes rather inconspicuous in H & E preparations, staining for alkaline phosphatase demonstrates it clearly (Figure 9.4).Its identification is important because the presence of a myoepithelial sheet co-extensive with the superficial layer of cells is valuable supporting evidence for the benignity of the lesion. Sometimes the fibrovascular stalks contain spaces lined by epithelium, producing a glandular appearance (Figures 9.5–9.7). Tumours with this pattern have been called papillary cystadenomas; the histological appearances can be confusing and may be misinterpreted as infiltrating carcinoma. This is particularly so if the glandular elements are closely opposed or, conversely, if there is a prominent fibrous stroma in which the epithelial structures are trapped (Figures 9.8–9.10). It can be especially misleading if the glandular elements extend into the stalk giving rise to an appearance of pseudo-infiltration of the duct wall (Figure 9.10). Another confusing pattern is produced by necrosis which can occur in both benign and malignant lesions (Figure 9.11). In patients with a heavily bloodstained discharge, thrombi may form in the ducts and subsequently become organized (Figure 9.12). Such a lesion should not be mistaken for a true papilloma, and

regarded as the definitive cause of a discharge.

An unusual pattern in a benign papilloma is illustrated in Figures 9.13 and 9.14. There is infiltration of the epithelial lining by pagetoid spread of carcinoma cells from a nearby *in situ* lobular carcinoma.

Papillary Carcinoma

In situ duct carcinoma may have a papillary pattern. Other patterns of *in situ* duct carcinoma are described in Chapter 10.

As mentioned above, the most significant discriminant between benign and malignant papillary lesions of the breast is the presence or absence of myoepithelium. Regular myoepithelial layers are absent from papillary carcinomas, whereas they are an important feature of benign papillomas. In papillary carcinomas, the malignant cells covering the fronds are usually only a few layers thick, but sometimes proliferation of the epithelial cells can produce solid or cribriform areas entirely lacking a papillary pattern. Although the cells may show obvious malignant characteristics with increased nuclear/cytoplasmic ratio, hyperchromasia and increased numbers of mitotic figures, the pattern is often strikingly monomorphic; this is partly due to the lack of myoepithelial layers. The presence of pink cell metaplasia is strongly indicative of benignity and is frequently seen in benign papillomas. In contrast to a benign papilloma, a papillary carcinoma usually has a much finer fibrovascular stalk, often with only thin-walled blood vessels and delicate collagen fibres (Figures 9.15 and 9.16). However, the amount of stroma varies considerably (Figures 9.17–9.20). The most helpful criteria in differentiating between benign and malignant papillomas have been clearly summarized by Kraus and Neubeker[2]. Similar criteria have been emphasized by Azzopardi[1]. However, as previously stressed, benign and malignant disease can coexist; for example, the neoplasm illustrated in Figures 9.21 and 9.22 appears to be a combination of a benign and malignant lesion within the same duct. But this must not be taken to indicate that solitary benign papillomas of the breast become carcinomas. On the other hand, there is evidence that the much rarer condition of multiple benign papillomas, which may extend well out into the breast from the subareolar region to involve an entire sector, is associated with an increased incidence of subsequent malignancy[3,4].

Intracystic Papillary Carcinoma

When an intraduct papillary carcinoma attains a sufficient size to present as a mass, the term 'intracystic

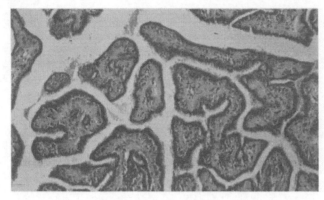

Figure 9.1 Intraduct papilloma. The branching fronds are cut in various planes, but all have well-formed fibrovascular cores covered by epithelium. The covering consists of a regular double cell layer: a row of juxtaluminal cuboidal cells and an underlying layer of myoepithelium.   H & E × 96

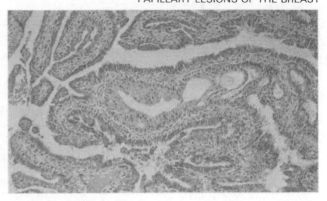

Figure 9.2 Intraduct papilloma: apocrine ('pink cell') metaplasia. The fronds are covered by typical double cell layers. In the middle of the field some of the epithelium shows 'pink cell' metaplasia.   H & E × 96

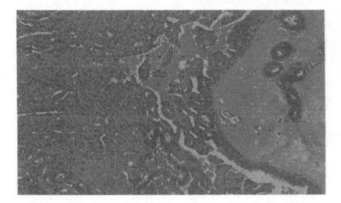

Figure 9.3 Intraduct papilloma. Although featuring a fronded pattern with double cell layers in some areas, other parts of this papilloma show the unusual cellular proliferative pattern illustrated here. The picture does not correspond with any of the recognized types of intraduct carcinoma, and is interpreted as pronounced epitheliosis arising in association with an intraduct papilloma. H & E × 96

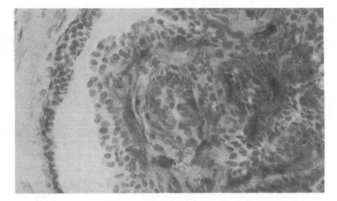

Figure 9.4 Intraduct papilloma: myoepithelial cells. The papilloma displays a prominent myoepithelial layer, stained red, beneath the juxtaluminal epithelium.   Azo coupling technique for alkaline phosphatase × 96

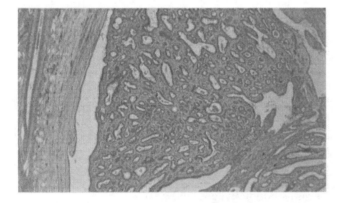

Figure 9.5 Intraduct papilloma. A lesion from the breast of a 14-year-old girl. In this example, the tumour forms a stalked mass protruding into the lumen of the duct and, instead of papillary projections, the epithelium forms tubules.   H & E × 24

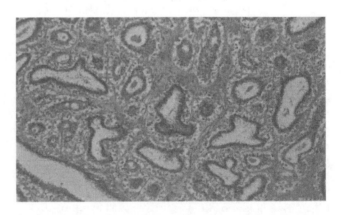

Figure 9.6 Intraduct papilloma. Higher magnification of the lesion shown in Figure 9.5. The tubules have distinct double cell layers and are supported by a fibrous stroma.   H & E × 96

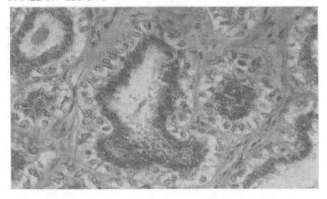

Figure 9.7 Intraduct papilloma. High-power view of the lesion illustrated in Figures 9.5 and 9.6. The myoepithelial cells display marked cytoplasmic vacuolation and form very obvious mantles around the juxtaluminal cells. H & E × 240

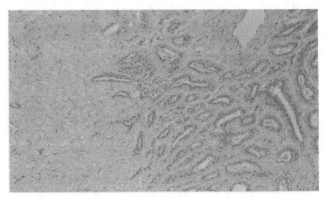

Figure 9.8 Sclerosing intraduct papilloma. An intraductal lesion with tubule formation and extensive sclerosis. In the left half of the field the epithelial structures have virtually disappeared and have been replaced by fibrous tissue. A spurious impression of invasion is produced, and such a lesion has to be distinguished from a tubular carcinoma. The presence of double cell layers and basement membranes around the tubules indicates benignity. H & E × 96

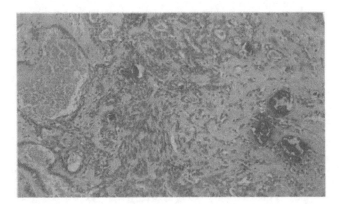

Figure 9.9 Sclerosing intraduct papilloma. Another sclerosing papillary lesion, featuring even greater distortion of the epithelium than that shown in Figure 9.8. There is also microcalcification. H & E × 96

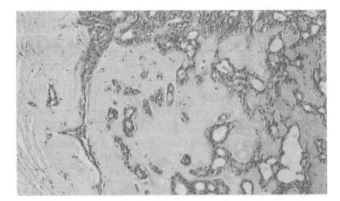

Figure 9.10 Sclerosing intraduct papilloma. Entrapment and distortion of tubules in dense hyaline fibrous tissue may be misinterpreted as invasive tumour. However, a double cell layer can be identified around many of the tubules, although the myoepithelium is attenuated and relatively inconspicuous. H & E × 96

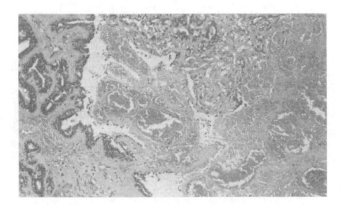

Figure 9.11 Intraduct papilloma with necrosis. The wall of the duct and some surrounding breast tissue is present on the left. The remainder of the field is occupied by the dilated duct lumen, containing mainly necrotic material and blood. A residuum of the papilloma can be recognized at the top centre of the photograph. H & E × 96

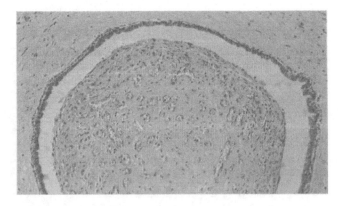

Figure 9.12 Intraductal granulation-tissue polyp. Section of a breast lesion in a woman who complained of bleeding from the nipple. The excised mammary tissue contained several intraductal polyps composed of vascular granulation tissue with very few inflammatory cells. The lining of the dilated duct is intact. The surface of the polyp has no epithelial covering. H & E × 96

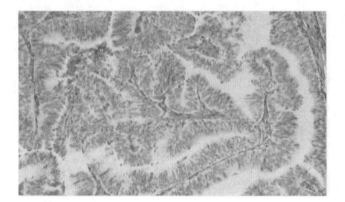

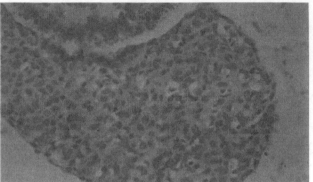

Figure 9.13 Intraduct papilloma with pagetoid change. Section of an intraduct papilloma which was situated in close proximity to foci of lobular carcinoma *in situ*. Several of the surrounding ducts showed pagetoid spread of carcinoma cells in their walls. In the illustration, pagetoid spread can be seen in the duct wall on the left. The club-shaped structure, lower centre, is a frond infiltrated and expanded by lobular carcinoma cells.   H & E × 96

Figure 9.14 Intraduct papilloma with pagetoid change. Higher magnifiction of the affected frond shown in Figure 9.13. The covering epithelium is attenuated, and the papilla is packed with numerous spheroidal lobular carcinoma cells.   H & E × 240

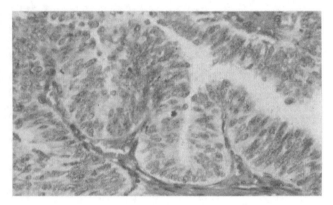

Figure 9.15 Papillary intraduct carcinoma. The fronds have very thin, vascular connective tissue septa, and are covered by epithelial cells piled up into several layers. The characteristic double cell layer of a benign papilloma is absent.   H & E × 96

Figure 9.16 Papillary intraduct carcinoma. Higher magnification of the lesion shown in Figure 9.15. Note the piling up of the epithelial cells into multiple layers, the presence of mitotic figures and the complete absence of a myoepithelial layer.   H & E × 240

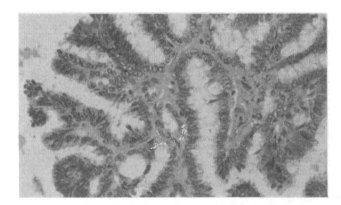

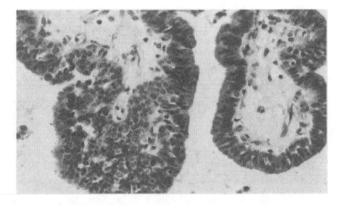

Figure 9.17 Papillary intraduct carcinoma. In this example the connective tissue cores are well formed and the covering epithelium is disposed as a single layer. All the epithelial cells are of one type: myoepithelium is absent. H & E × 240

Figure 9.18 Papillary intraduct carcinoma. Parts of two fronds with oedematous stroma covered by layers of hyperchromatic epithelial cells. Mitotic figures are present. The cells lying beneath the surface epithelium comprise capillary endothelial cells and other mesenchymal elements. Myoepithelium is completely absent.   H & E × 240

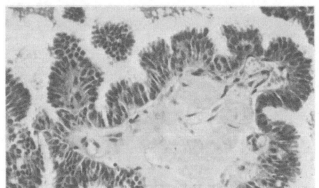

Figure 9.19 Papillary intraduct carcinoma. In this example, the fibrovascular cores of the papillae are thick and contain abundant collagen. The epithelial cells display stratification. There is no myoepithelial layer. H & E × 240

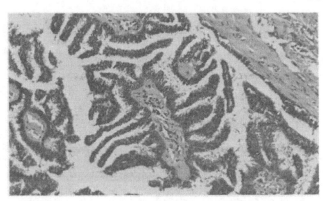

Figure 9.20 Papillary carcinoma. In this tumour the papillary processes have well-formed vascular fibrous cores covered by carcinoma cells which have proliferated to form long delicate fringes. Myoepithelial cells are absent. H & E × 96

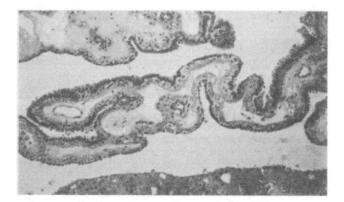

Figure 9.21 Intraduct papillary lesion with both benign and malignant components. Section of a papillary lesion from the breast of a 48-year-old woman. This photomicrograph shows a benign growth pattern. The frond running horizontally through the centre of the field displays a typical double cell layer, the myoepithelial cells being somewhat swollen and vacuolated. H & E × 96

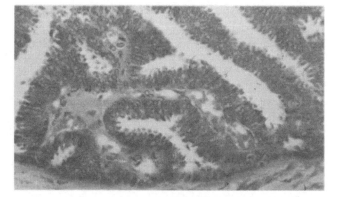

Figure 9.22 Intraduct papillary lesion with both benign and malignant components. Another part of the lesion illustrated in Figure 9.21. This shows a malignant papillary growth pattern: irregular stratification of the epithelial cells and no myoepithelial layer. H & E × 240

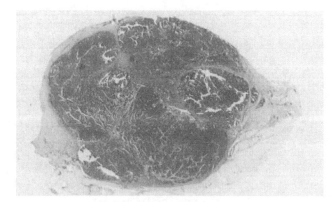

Figure 9.23 Intracystic papillary carcinoma. Section of a tumour from the breast of a 70-year-old woman. The neoplasm is sharply circumscribed, being surrounded by a fibrous capsule. The cyst is occupied by an intricate mass of branching fronds. H & E × 2.4

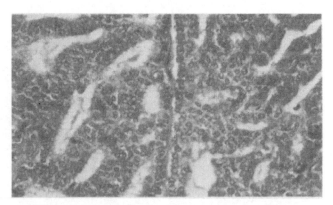

Figure 9.24 Intracystic papillary carcinoma. Photomicrograph of the tumour illustrated in Figure 9.23, showing the monomorphic cell pattern and complete absence of myoepithelium. The fronds with their thin connective tissue cores form a complex branching and anastomosing pattern. H & E × 240

papillary carcinoma' is usually applied (Figures 9.23 and 9.24). This type of carcinoma tends to occur in older women, usually over 50 years of age and with an average age approximately 10 years older than women with benign intraduct papillomas[5].

Careful examination of the wall of the duct or cyst is always necessary to exclude invasion in the case of a papillary carcinoma. Sometimes the papillary pattern is retained in the invasive component, and even in metastases, as described in Chapter 16, but more usually the invasive elements have the pattern of infiltrating duct carcinoma and are arranged in tubules or trabeculae.

References

1. Azzopardi, J. G. (1979). *Problems in Breast Pathology*, p. 150. (Vol. 11 in Bennington, J. L. (consulting ed.) *Major Problems in Pathology*.) (London, Philadelphia and Toronto: Saunders)
2. Kraus, F. T. and Neubecker, R. D. (1962). The differential diagnosis of papillary tumors of the breast. *Cancer*, **15**, 444
3. Haagensen, C. D., Bodian, C. and Haagensen, D. E. Jr. (1981). *Breast Carcinoma. Risk and Detection*, p. 197. (Philadelphia, London and Toronto: Saunders)
4. Murad, T. M., Contesso, G. and Mouriesse, H. (1981). Papillary tumors of large lactiferous ducts. *Cancer*. **48**, 122
5. Czernobilsky, B. (1967). Intracystic carcinoma of the female breast. *Surg. Gynecol. Obstet.*, **124**, 93

In situ duct carcinoma accounts for about 5% of all mammary carcinomas seen in general hospital practice. The incidence is higher in patients diagnosed in screening centres because the tumour is often detected by the presence of mammographic calcification in the absence of a palpable mass. Impalpable *in situ* duct carcinoma may also present as a nipple discharge, usually blood-stained, or as Paget's disease of the nipple. Residual tumour is frequently found in mastectomy specimens adjacent to the site of a biopsy containing *in situ* duct carcinoma, and true multicentric disease at a distance from the biopsy site can be demonstrated in about 30% of cases[1,2]. It is generally considered, however, that the incidence of multiple foci and of bilaterality is not so high with *in situ* duct carcinoma as with *in situ* lobular carcinoma.

There are various patterns of *in situ* duct carcinoma. The comedo type is probably the most common and is so called because on gross examination semi-solid material can be expressed from the dilated ducts. Microscopically the ducts are filled with pleomorphic malignant cells, often displaying many mitotic figures; there is necrosis in the centre of the cell masses and granular particles of calcium are frequently deposited in this area (Figures 10.1–10.3). In the less common solid type the lumen is entirely filled with malignant cells. The cribriform pattern is also seen quite frequently and may consist of an almost solid growth of malignant cells perforated by regular rounded spaces, or the lumen may be distended and the neoplastic cells form loops around the wall and bridges across the lumen (Figures 10.4–10.8). Calcification is also common in this type of *in situ* duct carcinoma but is usually psammomatous when present in the cribriform spaces. A combined cribriform and comedo pattern is not uncommon (Figure 10.3). *In situ* duct carcinoma with a papillary pattern is shown in Figure 10.9. Papillary fronds are covered by tall columnar cells which may be arranged in either single or multiple layers. There is no underlying myoepithelial layer and the supporting fibrovascular cores are usually thin and delicate. Marked expansion of the duct may occur in papillary *in situ* duct carcinoma with evolution to an intracystic papillary carcinoma. Differentiation of this type of tumour from benign papilloma has already been discussed (see Chapter 9). In the low papillary (micropapillary) pattern of *in situ* duct carcinoma no fibrovascular core is present, and the malignant cells form papillary tufts lining the duct (Figure 10.10). The malignant cells in cribriform and papillary *in situ* duct carcinoma tend to show less pleomorphism, with fewer mitotic figures than in the comedo and solid types. Occasionally *in situ* duct carcinoma is characterized by little or no obvious epithelial proliferation, although the cells lining the ducts have malignant characteristics; loss of polarity, increased

nuclear/cytoplasmic ratio, prominent nucleoli, nuclear hyperchromasia and increased numbers of mitotic figures with occasional abnormal mitoses (Figures 10.11 and 10.12). This type of tumour has been termed 'clinging carcinoma' by Azzopardi[3]. Some varieties probably represent comedo carcinoma in which most of the central necrotic debris within the duct has been lost, although others show no evidence of such an evolution. More than one pattern of *in situ* duct carcinoma is often present within the same lesion (Figure 10.13).

Spread of *in situ* duct carcinoma into lobular acini has been termed 'cancerization of lobules'. In general, the lobular architecture is retained but the acini are filled and distended by the malignant cells (Figures 10.14–10.16). This condition must be distinguished from lobular carcinoma *in situ*[4]. In lobular cancerization, the malignant cells are larger and more pleomorphic than the rather regular cells of lobular carcinoma *in situ*. Furthermore, the pattern of the carcinoma within the cancerized lobules usually resembles that of conventional *in situ* duct carcinoma with a comedo, solid or cribriform structure and intraduct carcinoma of a similar pattern is frequently present in the surrounding breast. Although cancerization of lobules can usually be distinguished from *in situ* lobular carcinoma without difficulty, occasionally differentiation between the two is not possible. As well as spreading into lobules, *in situ* duct carcinoma may extend along the ducts in a pagetoid fashion, a phenomenon more commonly associated with *in situ* lobular carcinoma (Figure 10.17). In many sections of *in situ* duct carcinoma, myoepithelial cells can still be identified around the duct; however, these are often stretched and attenuated and rarely, if ever, show evidence of proliferation (Figure 10.18). By contrast, benign intraductal hyperplasia usually features proliferation, both of myoepithelial cells and the juxta-luminal cells, as mentioned and illustrated in Chapter 5, where the differentiation of benign hyperplastic lesions from *in situ* carcinoma is discussed in more detail.

All cases of *in situ* duct carcinoma should be carefully examined for evidence of infiltration. Multiple blocks and multiple levels of each block must be scrutinized. The presence of prominent stromal elastosis should prompt a particularly careful search because, according to some authorities, this often indicates that invasion has occurred[3]. Rosen *et al.*[2] found that when *in situ* duct carcinoma was diagnosed at frozen section, invasive carcinoma was detected after wider sampling of the biopsy specimen in 20% of the cases, and even when no invasion was seen in the biopsy specimen, infiltrating carcinoma was found in the mastectomy specimen in a further 6% of cases. This is lower than the 21% incidence of occult invasive carcinoma reported by Lagios *et al.*[1]. They found that the incidence of occult foci of invasion and multicentric *in situ* change was

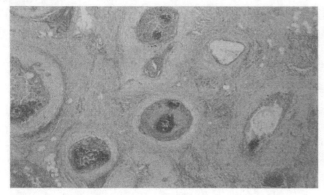

Figure 10.1 Comedo carcinoma of the breast. Section of a mammary tumour which was predominantly intraductal. In this field, the duct walls are thickened and their lumina distended with malignant cells. Central necrosis and dystrophic calcification has occurred in many of the ducts. H & E × 24

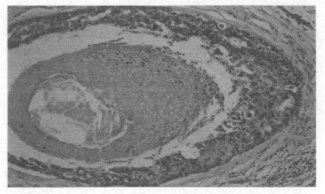

Figure 10.2 Intraduct carcinoma, comedo type. Section showing a distended duct with viable, pleomorphic carcinoma cells at the periphery. Centrally, extensive coagulative necrosis has occurred, and there is a mass of amorphous eosinophilic material containing pyknotic nuclear remnants. H & E × 240

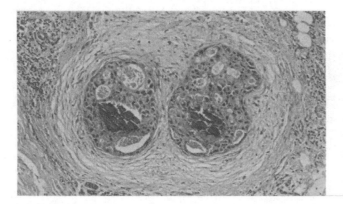

Figure 10.3 Intraduct carcinoma with comedo and cribriform patterns. The walls of the ducts are thickened and the lumina contains pleomorphic carcinoma cells. Both cribriform and comedo patterns are apparent, the necrotic material being calcified and staining blue with haematoxylin. H & E × 96

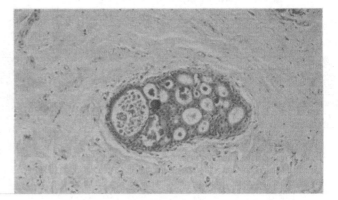

Figure 10.4 Intraduct carcinoma, cribriform type, with calcification. The section shows a duct with a typical cribriform carcinoma *in situ*. The material in the spaces has undergone calcification and appears as rounded and irregularly shaped haematoxyphil bodies. H & E × 96

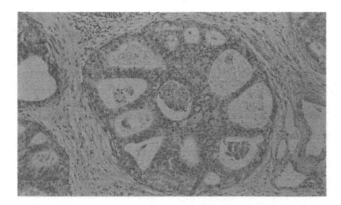

Figure 10.5 Intraduct carcinoma, cribriform type. An example of the so-called 'cartwheel' pattern: columns of tumour cells, between the cribriform spaces, tend to be arranged radially in a manner reminiscent of the spokes of a wheel. H & E × 96

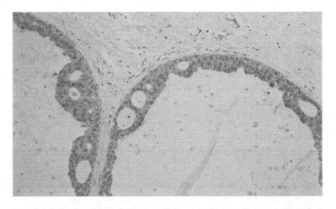

Figure 10.6 Intraduct carcinoma, cribriform type. The ducts are distended and contain some proteinaceous coagulum. The carcinoma cells are confined to the periphery where they form loops. There is no supporting stroma amongst the tumour cells. H & E × 96

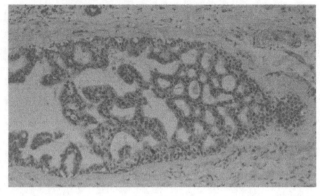

Figure 10.7 Intraduct carcinoma, cribriform type. On the right a typical cribriform pattern is seen: elsewhere the cells form peripheral loops and irregular sinuous projections into the lumen. The proliferating cells lack a supporting stroma.   H & E × 96

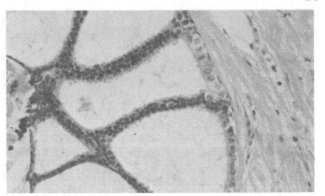

Figure 10.8 Intraduct carcinoma, cribriform type. Another example in which the bridging cell-columns tend to form a radial pattern. Note that the nuclei are fairly regular in size, shape and staining properties, and that the bridge lacks a supporting stroma.   H & E × 240

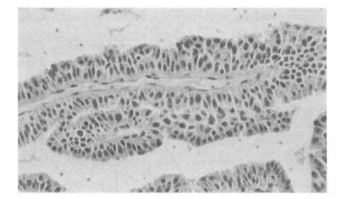

Figure 10.9 Intraduct carcinoma, papillary type. Part of a papillary frond within the lumen of a distended duct. The frond has a delicate vascular core, comprising little more than a thin-walled capillary blood vessel; the single layer of endothelial cells can be seen clearly. The tumour cells are piled up in an irregular array, and there is no evidence of a myoepithelial mantle. H & E × 240

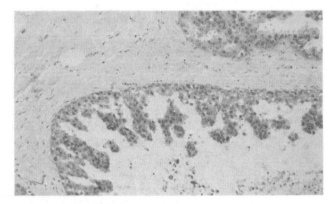

Figure 10.10 Intraduct carcinoma, low papillary type. The duct is dilated, but the neoplastic cells are confined to the periphery where they form an irregular fringe. They display neither a cribriform nor a true papillary pattern. True papillary carcinoma is characterized by dichotomous branching and by connective tissue cores supporting the fronds.   H & E × 96

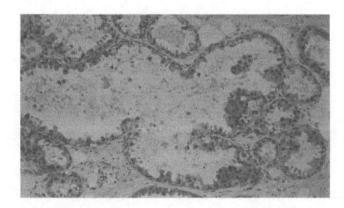

Figure 10.11 Intraduct carcinoma, 'clinging' and low papillary patterns. The ducts are dilated and contain a few degenerate cells within a predominantly fluid content. Pleomorphic carcinoma cells are adherent to the inner surface of the wall; they are mostly devoid of any special arrangement, but a small papillary ingrowth is present on the right.   H & E × 96

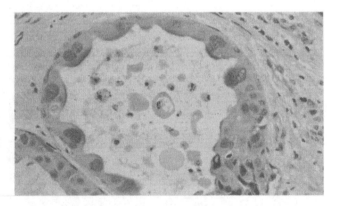

Figure 10.12 Intraduct carcinoma, 'clinging' type. The lumen of the duct is distended and contains a few degenerate cells with karyorrhectic nuclear remnants. There is a peripheral layer of carcinoma cells displaying abundant amphophilic cytoplasm and large pleomorphic nuclei.   H & E × 240

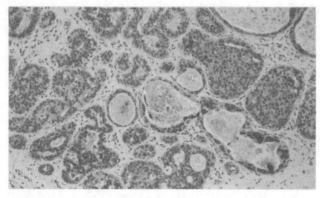

Figure 10.13 Intraduct carcinoma, mixed pattern. This tumour displays a combination of solid and 'clinging' carcinoma. At the bottom centre of the field there is also a suggestion of a cribriform pattern. Many of the cells are fairly regular, but large, bizarre, hyperchromatic forms are present in the 'clinging' carcinoma towards the lower right hand corner of the photograph. H & E × 96

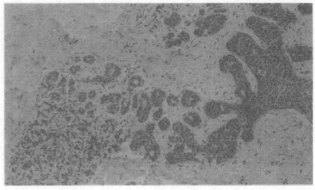

Figure 10.14 Extension of intraduct carcinoma into lobule. An example of so-called 'cancerization' of a lobule. On the right, there is a branching duct filled with pleomorphic carcinoma cells. The ramification of this duct, and its cellular content, can be traced to the lobule in the lower left-hand corner of the field. H & E × 96

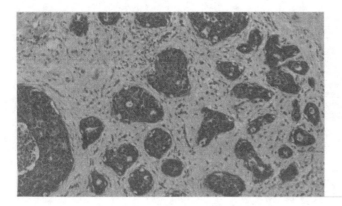

Figure 10.15 Extension of intraduct carcinoma into lobule. Most of the field is occupied by a mammary lobule as shown by its circular outline and loose stroma. At the bottom left-hand corner, there is part of a duct filled with carcinoma cells. The large, pleomorphic cells of the duct carcinoma have spread into the lobule to fill and distend the ductules and acini. H & E × 96

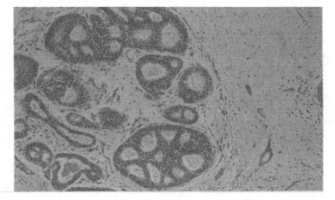

Figure 10.16 Extension of intraduct carcinoma into lobule. The lobule in the left half of the field shows marked distension of its ductules and acini by cribriform carcinoma which has extended in from an adjacent duct. H & E × 240

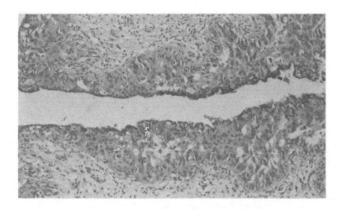

Figure 10.17 Pagetoid spread of duct carcinoma into wall of adjacent duct. Pagetoid extension along duct walls is usually secondary to lobular carcinoma. Occasionally duct carcinoma spreads in a similar fashion as shown here. A zone of large pleomorphic tumour cells is present between the outer wall of the duct and the attenuated layer of lining cells adjacent to the lumen. Compare the cytological features with those of the lesion illustrated in previous figures. H & E × 96

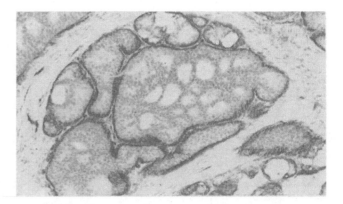

Figure 10.18 Intraduct carcinoma, cribriform type. Photomicrograph showing a frozen section of unfixed tissue stained for alkaline phosphatase. Myoepithelial cells, stained red, are still present in the walls of the ducts, but they have not proliferated *pari passu* with the tumour cells, in contrast to their behaviour in benign intraduct lesions such as papillomas. Azo coupling technique for alkaline phosphatase × 96

related to size and was significantly higher in patients whose presenting lesions measured 2.5 cm or more.

Even when no invasion can be identified by light microscopy, electron microscopy will demonstrate small foci of malignant cells protruding through the basal lamina in most cases[5]. The difficulty of excluding invasion is further illustrated by the fact that approximately 1–2% of patients thought to have pure *in situ* duct carcinoma are found at mastectomy to have secondary deposits in axillary lymph nodes[1,2]. Conversely, occasional patients present with axillary lymph node metastases in whom only *in situ* duct carcinoma can be found at mastectomy[6].

Recently there have been several reports of patients with pure *in situ* duct carcinoma treated by biopsy alone: the incidence of subsequent invasive carcinoma has varied from 28% to 50%[7–9]. The invasive tumours all developed in the ipsilateral breast, on average 10 years after the date of the biopsy[8], in contrast to patients with *in situ* lobular carcinoma who suffer an increased risk of cancer subsequently developing in either breast after an average 20 year interval.

References

1. Lagios, M. D., Westdahl, P. R., Margolin, F. R. and Rose, M. R. (1982). Duct carcinoma in situ. Relationship of extent of non-invasive disease to the frequency of occult invasion, multi-centricity, lymph-node metastases and short-term treatment failures. *Cancer*, **50**, 1309

2. Rosen, P. P., Senie, R., Schottenfeld, D. and Ashikari, R. (1979). Noninvasive breast carcinoma. Frequency of unsuspected invasion and implications for treatment. *Ann. Surg.* **189**, 377

3. Azzopardi, J. G. (1979). *Problems in Breast Pathology*, p. 193. (Vol. 11 in Bennington, J. L. (consulting ed.) *Major Problems in Pathology*.) (London, Philadelphia and Toronto: Saunders)

4. Fechner, R. E. (1971). Ductal carcinoma involving the lobule of the breast. *Cancer*, **28**, 274

5. Ozzello, L. (1971). Ultrastructure of intra-epithelial carcinomas of the breast. *Cancer*, **28**, 1508

6. Rosen, P. P. (1980). Axillary lymph node metastases in patients with occult noninvasive breast carcinoma. *Cancer*, **46**, 1298

7. Betsill, W. L., Rosen, P. P., Lieberman, P. H. and Robbins, G. F. (1978). Intraductal carcinoma. Long-term follow-up after treatment by biopsy alone. *J. Am. Med. Assoc.*, **239**, 1863

8. Page, D. L., Dupont, W. D., Rogers, L. W. and Landenberger, M. (1982). Intraductal carcinoma of the breast: follow-up after biopsy only. *Cancer*, **49**, 751

9. Rosen, P. P., Braun, D. W. and Kinne, D. E. (1980). The clinical significance of pre-invasive breast carcinoma. *Cancer*, **46**, 919

In Situ Lobular Carcinoma

Lobular carcinoma *in situ* was first described as a distinct entity by Foote and Stewart in 1941[1], although there is still considerable controversy concerning the true nature of the lesion and the most appropriate terminology. Haagensen and colleagues[2] consider the lesion to be precancerous and call it simply 'lobular neoplasia', while Toker and Goldberg[3] prefer the noncommittal term '*in situ* small cell lesion'. It is usually an incidental finding in biopsies performed for other reasons, such as cystic disease, since it does not itself produce a palpable mass and it cannot be recognized macroscopically. Although lobular carcinoma *in situ* is sometimes found in tissue removed because of mammographic calcification, it is rare for the calcium deposits actually to be within the tumour foci; they are usually situated in adjacent non-neoplastic tissue. Pure lobular carcinoma *in situ* accounts for about 2–3% of all mammary carcinomas. Discrepancies in the incidence reported in the literature may be attributable to geographical variations as well as to different diagnostic criteria and thoroughness of examination of breast biopsy tissue. Lobular carcinoma shows a high incidence of multicentricity and bilaterality. Multicentricity has been estimated to be at least 70% and bilaterality at least 30–35%[4].

Approximately three quarters of women with pure lobular carcinoma *in situ* are premenopausal, with an average age of 45 years. Lobular carcinoma *in situ* has not been described in males.

There is no characteristic gross appearance but the lesion is frequently found in association with cystic disease. The histological features are illustrated in Figures 11.1–11.5. The overall architecture of the lobules is retained but the individual acini are distended by neoplastic cells which usually, but not always, completely fill the lumen, are evenly spaced, lack cohesion and are arranged in a loose and random fashion. The involved acini stand out in marked contrast to those of the adjacent normal lobules. It is worth emphasizing that good fixation of tissue is particularly important in the diagnosis of lobular carcinoma *in situ*; imperfect fixation and processing can result in artefacts leading to an erroneous diagnosis[5]. Likewise, diagnosis of lobular carcinoma *in situ* on frozen section can be extremely difficult; furthermore, the material may not include the lesion as there is no characteristic gross appearance to aid selection. The cytological features are often strikingly uniform; the tumour cells are smaller than in duct carcinoma, although larger than normal cells, and are quite regular in size and staining properties, with rounded to oval nuclei, inconspicuous nucleoli and few mitotic figures (Figures 11.1, 11.2 and 11.4). In some cases the cells are both slightly larger and show more variation in size and shape (Figures 11.3 and 11.5). In early descriptions Haagensen and colleagues

called this 'type B' and named the uniform pattern 'type A', but they have since abandoned this classification and consider there is a continuous spectrum of appearances[2]. Single lobules or several lobules may be involved and occasionally only part of an individual lobule is affected. There is also variation in the degree to which the acini are distended; occasionally they are markedly expanded and closely opposed. Mucin stains reveal cytoplasmic globules in many of the cells in most, but not all, cases of lobular carcinoma *in situ* (Figure 11.6). Granular mucin is less common. The globules contain alcianophilic haloes and often a central core of neutral muco-substance producing a 'target' or 'bull's-eye' appearance, with the combined Alcian blue/PAS stain (Figure 11.7). This characteristic appearance is considered by some authorities to be helpful in distinguishing between lobular carcinoma *in situ* and cancerization of lobules by intraduct carcinoma[6].

Just as *in situ* duct carcinoma can extend into lobules, so *in situ* lobular carcinoma may extend into the small ducts. The tumour cells often infiltrate the duct walls to produce the pagetoid appearance shown in Figures 11.8 and 11.9. When this process is extensive it may result in the clover leaf pattern shown in Figure 11.10. Sometimes pagetoid infiltration of the ducts is the only abnormality seen in the initial sections of a biopsy, and its appearance should prompt further search for associated lobular carcinoma *in situ*. In postmenopausal women the ductal phase may be more conspicuous because of involution of the lobules. A pattern of pseudo-pagetoid spread may be produced by the presence of vacuolated cells, probably histiocytes, within the duct walls (Figure 11.11). This must be distinguished from the pagetoid spread associated with lobular carcinoma *in situ*. Solid papillary and cribriform patterns of spread into adjacent ducts have also been described[7] and are shown in Figures 11.12 and 11.13. Sometimes the ducts, which are entirely filled with neoplastic cells, show central necrosis, and the lesion may simulate intraduct carcinoma of comedo type (Figure 11.14). Indeed, it is argued by some that such a picture represents *in situ* duct carcinoma mimicking *in situ* lobular carcinoma, rather than true ductal spread of *in situ* lobular carcinoma[2].

The differential diagnosis of lobular carcinoma *in situ* includes benign hyperplasia on the one hand, and *in situ* duct carcinoma or infiltrating carcinoma on the other. Atypical lobular hyperplasia, as already described in Chapter 5, shows some of the features of lobular carcinoma *in situ*, but does not fulfill all the criteria (Figures 11.15 and 11.16). There is only partial lobular involvement with less distension of the acini and some persistence of the lumina. The proliferating cells are less uniform than those of lobular carcinoma *in situ*, and they are crowded together without the lack of cohesion

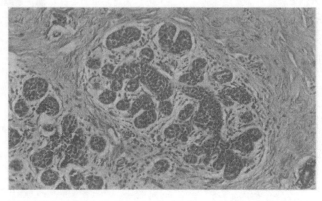

Figure 11.1 Lobular carcinoma *in situ*. The ductules and acini of the lobule are distended with loosely arranged, darkly-staining, uniform spheroidal tumour cells, and the lumina are obliterated.   H & E × 96

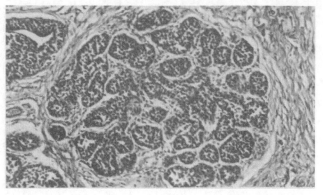

Figure 11.2 Lobular carcinoma *in situ*. In this example the whole lobule is somewhat enlarged by the prominence and generalized distension of the ductules and acini by the tumour cells. The cells are relatively small, deeply stained with haematoxylin and lack cohesion. The lumina have been effaced.   H & E × 96

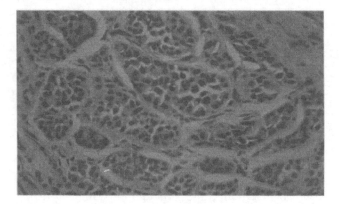

Figure 11.3 Lobular carcinoma *in situ*. A high-power view showing the loosely arranged, hyperchromatic carcinoma cells, filling and distending the acini. In this example the tumour cells are slightly larger and more pleomorphic in contrast to the 'small-cell' type shown in Figures 11.1 and 11.2.   H & E × 240

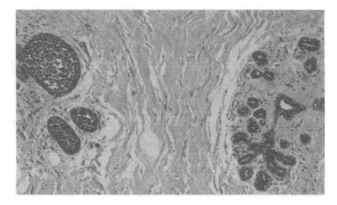

Figure 11.4 Lobular carcinoma *in situ*. Photomicrograph contrasting the ductules of the normal lobule on the right with those distended by darkly-staining carcinoma cells on the left.   H & E × 96

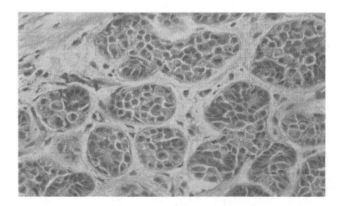

Figure 11.5 Lobular carcinoma *in situ*. A high-power view of an affected lobule. In this example the cells have more abundant cytoplasm which is somewhat vacuolated. Special stains reveal abundant intracytoplasmic mucin.   H & E × 240

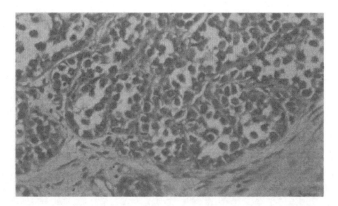

Figure 11.6 Lobular carcinoma *in situ*. Section illustrating abundant mucin in the cytoplasm of the tumour cells. The mucin stains bright red.   PAS after diastase digestion × 240

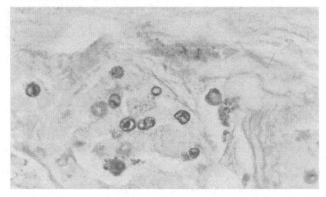

Figure 11.7 Lobular carcinoma *in situ*. Section stained to show intracyto-plasmic globules of mucin present in some of the cells. The combined Alcian blue/PAS stain shows the characteristic target or bull's-eye pattern of staining with a dark blue peripheral ring and central core.   Combined Alcian blue/PAS × 240

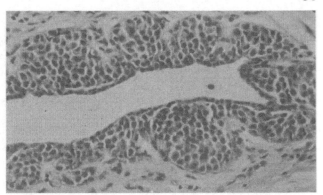

Figure 11.8 Lobular carcinoma *in situ*: pagetoid spread in wall of a duct. Section of a duct from the neighbourhood of an intralobular carcinoma. Darkly-staining, spheroidal tumour cells have infiltrated the duct wall between the attenuated layer of juxtaluminal cells and the basement membrane. H & E × 240

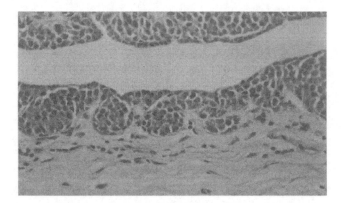

Figure 11.9 Lobular carcinoma *in situ*: pagetoid spread in wall of a duct. From the same lesion as that illustrated in Figure 11.8. The section has been stained to show the intracytoplasmic mucin (coloured red) of the tumour cells.   PAS after diastase digestion × 240

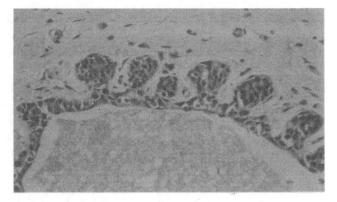

Figure 11.10 Lobular carcinoma *in situ*: pagetoid spread in wall of a duct. Another configuration in which the infiltrating tumour cells form a bead-like pattern around the periphery of the duct.   H & E × 240

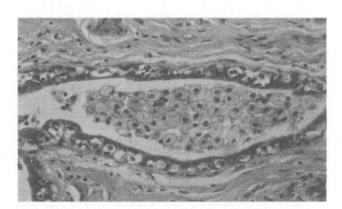

Figure 11.11 Pseudo-pagetoid change in wall of a duct. The wall contains vacuolated cells, probably histiocytes, and cells with abundant foamy cytoplasm are present in the lumen. No lobular carcinoma could be found in the adjacent breast, and no mucin could be demonstrated in the cells within the duct wall.   H & E × 240

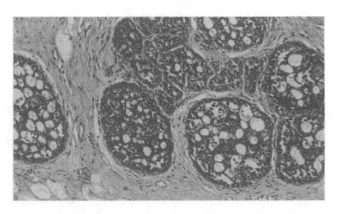

Figure 11.12 Lobular carcinoma *in situ*. The ductules and acini are greatly dis-tended by the darkly-staining tumour cells which are arranged so as to form a cribriform carcinoma, but the small spheroidal cells seen here are charac-teristic of lobular carcinoma.   H & E × 96

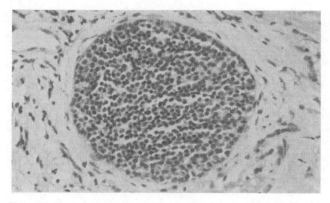

Figure 11.13 Lobular carcinoma. This photomicrograph shows a duct filled and distended by cells characteristic of lobular carcinoma of small-cell type. In this field there is also infiltration of the stroma by carcinoma cells. H & E × 240

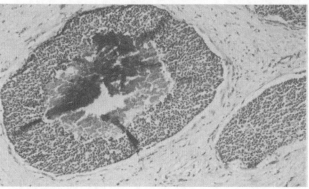

Figure 11.14 Lobular carcinoma *in situ*. The tumour cells have distended medium-sized ducts and extensive necrosis has occurred centrally, producing a 'comedo' pattern. Such a pattern is much more common in intraduct carcinoma, but again the small spheroidal cells are characteristic of lobular carcinoma. H & E × 96

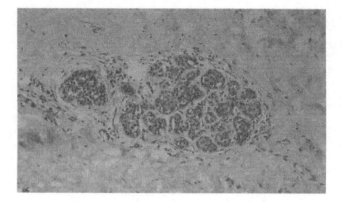

Figure 11.15 Atypical lobular hyperplasia. Hyperplastic epithelial cells are present in the ductules and acini, but they do not completely obliterate the lumina. This is a controversial lesion which some workers regard as an early stage in the development of lobular neoplasia. H & E × 96

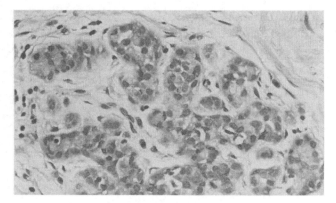

Figure 11.16 Atypical lobular hyperplasia. A high-power view of the lesion illustrated in Figure 11.15. The hyperplastic cells do not completely obliterate the lumina of the acini nor do they display the lack of cohesion so characteristic of lobular carcinoma cells. H & E × 240

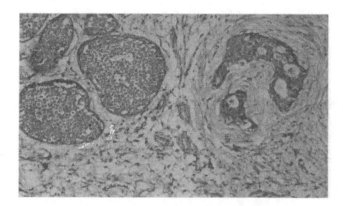

Figure 11.17 Combined lobular and intraduct carcinoma. In the left half of the field there are ductules distended with uniform spheroidal cells typical of *in situ* lobular carcinoma. On the right a ductule contains larger and more pleomorphic cells, arranged in a cribriform pattern; an intraduct carcinoma. H & E × 96

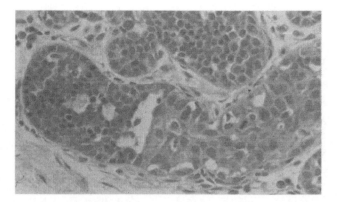

Figure 11.18 Combined lobular and intraduct carcinoma involving the same lobular ductal unit. In this single unit on the left, the acinus is distended with uniform spheroidal cells characteristic of lobular carcinoma *in situ*, whilst on the right the proliferating cells are larger and more pleomorphic and resemble those seen in duct carcinoma *in situ*. H & E × 240

so typical of lobular carcinoma *in situ*. As mentioned, this change is frequent in breasts in which fully developed *in situ* or infiltrating lobular carcinoma is present elsewhere. Cancerization of the lobules by *in situ* duct carcinoma is best distinguished by the cytological characteristics of the malignant cells, which show much more pleomorphism, and by the fact that the pattern within the acini often resembles that in the surrounding ducts, featuring the well-recognizable comedo, cribriform or solid configurations[8]. Although distinction between the two usually presents no problem, differential diagnosis is sometimes extremely difficult or impossible. Furthermore, *in situ* lobular carcinoma and *in situ* duct carcinoma can occur side by side (Figure 11.17) or involve the same lobular ductal unit (Figure 11.18).

As in all cases of *in situ* carcinoma, careful examination of tissue containing lobular carcinoma *in situ* must be made in order to exclude invasion. A confusing pattern mimicking invasion can be produced when sclerosing adenosis affects lobules involved with lobular carcinoma *in situ*[9]. The risk of occult invasive carcinoma elsewhere in the breast is relatively low. Rosen *et al.*[10] found invasive carcinoma in the mastectomy specimen of 4% of patients in whom only lobular carcinoma *in situ* was seen in the biopsy specimen. When infiltrating carcinoma is present in association with *in situ* lobular carcinoma, although it is of lobular type in about 50% of cases, the invasive growth may be of ductal type.

Follow-up studies of patients with lobular carcinoma *in situ* treated by biopsy alone show an increased incidence of subsequent invasive carcinoma. The reported risk varies from 16 to 27%[11]. In two large recent studies the incidence was found to be seven times greater than expected in the general population in one study[2], and nine times greater in the other[11]. In the latter study mortality from mammary carcinoma was eleven times greater than expected. The hazard increases with increasing age and length of follow-up. In the study by Rosen *et al.*[11], whose report includes patients with the longest average follow-up, the majority of subsequent carcinomas became evident 15 or more years after the original biopsy and 38% were not detected until 20 years had elapsed. The subsequent carcinoma may occur within either the ipsi- or contralateral breast and may be of either ductal or lobular type. Although some authorities have found that subsequent carcinomas tend to be those associated with a more favourable prognosis than average[2], other studies have not substantiated this[11]. There are apparently no special histological features which help predict which particular women with lobular carcinoma *in situ* are at most risk of subsequent carcinoma. Haagensen *et al.*[2] have found that the risk is increased in women with coexistent cystic disease particularly if there is also a family history of breast cancer. No such correlation has been noted by others[11].

References

1. Foote, F. W. Jr. and Stewart, F. W. (1941). Lobular carcinoma in situ. *Am. J. Pathol.*, **17**, 491

2. Haagensen, C. D., Lane, N., Lattes, R. and Bodian, C. (1978). Lobular neoplasia (so-called lobular carcinoma in situ) of the breast. *Cancer*, **42**, 737

3. Toker, C. and Goldberg, J. D. (1977). The small cell lesion of mammary ducts and lobules. In Sommers, S. C. and Rosen, P. P. (eds.) *Pathology Annual*, Vol. 12, pp. 217–249. (New York: Appleton-Century-Crofts)

4. Andersen, J. A. and Schiodt, T. (1980). On the concept of carcinoma in situ of the breast. *Pathol. Res. Pract.*, **166**, 407

5. Wheeler, J. E. and Enterline, H. T. (1976). Lobular carcinoma of the breast in situ and infiltrating. In Sommers, S. C. (ed.) *Pathology Annual*, Vol. 11, pp. 161–188, (New York: Appleton-Century-Crofts)

6. Andersen, J. A. and Vendleboe, M. L. (1981). Cytoplasmic mucous globules in lobular carcinoma in situ. *Am. J. Surg. Pathol.*, **5**, 251

7. Fechner, R. E. and Houston, M. D. (1972). Epithelial alterations in the extralobular ducts of breasts with lobular carcinoma. *Arch. Pathol.*, **93**, 164

8. Fechner, R. E. (1971). Ductal carcinoma involving the lobule of the breast. *Cancer*, **28**, 274

9. Fechner, R. E. (1981). Lobular carcinoma in situ in sclerosing adenosis. *Am. J. Surg. Pathol.*, **5**, 233

10. Rosen, P. P., Senie, R., Schottenfeld, D. and Ashikari, R. (1979). Noninvasive breast carcinoma. Frequency of unsuspected invasion and implications for treatment. *Ann. Surg.*, **189**, 377

11. Rosen, P. P., Lieberman, P. H., Braun, D. W. Jr., Kosloff, C. and Adair, F. (1978). Lobular carcinoma in situ of the breast. *Am. J. Surg. Pathol.*, **2**, 225

Infiltrating duct carcinomas comprise the majority of invasive cancers and most of the tumours are depicted without special features, or not otherwise specified (NOS)[1]. Some workers divide these tumours into (1) stellate carcinomas with productive fibrosis and (2) circumscribed or multinodular carcinomas[2].

Stellate carcinomas contain a large amount of dense hyaline stroma which imparts a very firm consistency to the growth – hence the old term 'scirrhous carcinoma'. At low magnification sections of such neoplasms demonstrate their irregular outline, with tentacles of tumour extending into the surrounding breast and drawing adjacent tissue inwards towards the neoplasm (Figure 12.1). The stroma often contains a very large amount of elastic tissue appearing macroscopically as yellowish streaks on the cut surface (Figure 12.2).

Circumscribed or multinodular carcinomas have a well-defined rounded or lobulated edge (Figure 12.3). This has sometimes been described as a 'pushing' border. Such tumours are usually more cellular than the stellate carcinomas and the stroma is very often loose and fibrovascular. However, some tumours with this type of outline have a cellular periphery and a very densely fibrotic centre.

Various systems for grading infiltrating duct carcinomas have been devised. The one most commonly used in the UK is that of Bloom and Richardson[3], in which three grades are described. The system is based on three microscopic features: tubular differentiation, the degree of nuclear pleomorphism and the number of mitotic figures. Each feature is scored from 1 to 3 and the digits are summed, giving a total within the range of 3 to 9 points. Tumours scoring 3, 4 and 5 are classified as Grade I, well-differentiated tumours; those scoring 6 and 7 are Grade II, moderately differentiated tumours; and those scoring 8 and 9 are poorly differentiated, Grade III tumours. The middle Grade II category usually accounts for at least half the total number. Of the remaining neoplasms two thirds usually fit into Grade III and one third into Grade I. Although there is a significant correlation between grade and prognosis in respect of Grade I tumours, the prognostic difference between Grade II and III tumours appears to be lost after 10 years and with a further lapse of time the difference between all three grades becomes less significant. Moreover, the small number of tumours falling into the Grade I category somewhat detracts from the value of this system. There are various modifications of the grading system. In some, different levels of significance are placed on the various scoring factors.

There is considerable variation in the microscopic features of infiltrating duct carcinoma NOS and it is not possible to illustrate fully even the most common patterns. Well-differentiated (Grade I) tumours as shown in Figure 12.4 are composed of fairly uniform cells with a low mitotic rate and a tubular arrangement. Figures 12.5 and 12.6 show transitions between such a Grade I tumour and the very poorly differentiated Grade III tumour shown in Figures 12.7 and 12.8. Between the Grade I and Grade III tumours there is a progressive increase in cellular and nuclear pleomorphism and in the number of mitotic figures. In the tumour illustrated in Figure 12.7, abnormal mitoses are also present. In poorly differentiated carcinomas, the tubular growth pattern is replaced by trabeculae and clumps of neoplastic cells. The size of the clumps varies considerably, from clusters of 3–5 cells to large masses in which foci of necrosis may be present. Although most carcinomas are fairly uniform in the appearance and pattern of the malignant cells, some show considerable variation from area to area. Rarely, carcinoma of the breast may show spindle-cell dedifferentiation and the microscopic appearance mimics a sarcoma. Careful search, however, will usually reveal a transition between the spindle-shaped sarcomatoid cells and the more conventional carcinoma cells (Figures 12.9 and 12.10). In some tumours the malignant cells may be very pleomorphic and bizarre and tumour giant cells can occur (Figure 12.11).

The amount of mucin within the malignant cells is very variable; it is often present within the lumen of the tubules but is sometimes intracellular, although the latter is more common in lobular carcinoma. Occasional cells of signet-ring type may be present but these are also more frequently associated with infiltrating lobular carcinoma. Pure signet-ring carcinomas are best classified as a separate tumour type (see Chapter 15).

Metaplastic changes in the malignant cells can produce a variety of patterns, many of which are considered later in Chapter 16. Apocrine metaplasia of the malignant cells is not uncommon but pure apocrine tumours are rare. Squamous metaplasia or cells with a squamoid appearance are also common, but again pure squamous cell carcinoma of the breast is extremely uncommon. Very rarely chondroid or osseous metaplasia is seen. Carcinomas showing these various metaplastic changes are sometimes designated as separate tumour types but, as their prognostic significance in most cases is uncertain, there seems to be little clinical value in so doing.

As already mentioned, the amount and nature of the stroma also vary considerably. The dense hyaline stroma shown in Figure 12.12 contains only a few malignant cells and difficulty may be experienced in distinguishing a small tumour with this pattern from sclerosing adenosis. In some tumours the stroma, although abundant, is more cellular (Figure 12.13), and in others it is extremely sparse (Figure 12.14). Sometimes the stroma is rich in connective tissue mucin as shown in Figures 12.15 and 12.16. Occasionally osteo-

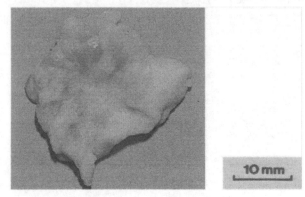

Figure 12.1 Infiltrating duct carcinoma with stellate outline. The tumour has a dense fibrous stroma, and there is prominent periductal elastosis (the elastic staining black in this preparation). Fibrous trabeculae radiate outwards from the main mass, and the limits of the growth are ill-defined.   Verhoeff elastic stain/van Gieson × 2.4

Figure 12.2 Infiltrating duct carcinoma with productive fibrosis ('scirrhous carcinoma'). Cut surface of a bisected gross specimen showing the lack of encapsulation, the stellate outline, the contracted (concave) surface and the thin yellow streaks of elastosis within the tumour

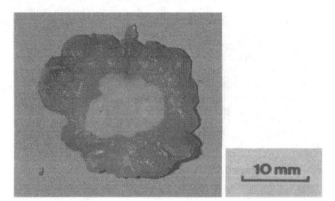

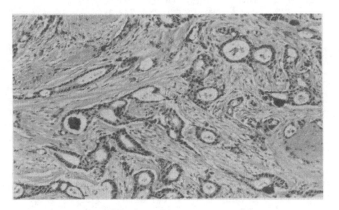

Figure 12.3 Infiltrating duct carcinoma with circumscribed outline. The cut surface of a bisected gross specimen showing the circumscribed 'pushing' outline and the contracted (concave) surface. The tumour is clearly demarcated from the surrounding fat

Figure 12.4 Infiltrating duct carcinoma, well-differentiated (Grade I). Section of a tumour featuring prominent tubular differentiation. Many of the tubules comprise only a single layer of cells and mitotic figures are extremely sparse. There is a moderately abundant fibroblastic stroma. A few foci of microcalcification are present.   H & E × 96

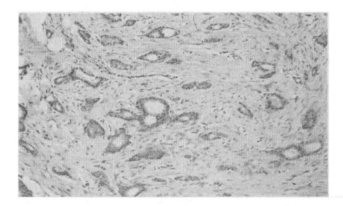

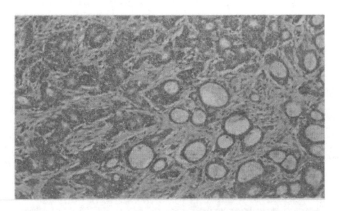

Figure 12.5 Infiltrating duct carcinoma (Grade II). This is a tumour of average grade malignancy, featuring prominent tubular differentiation. The stroma is moderately cellular and displays definite collagen formation; but it lacks the density, the abundance of collagen and parvicellular character of a typical 'scirrhous' carcinoma.   H & E × 96

Figure 12.6 Infiltrating duct carcinoma (Grade II). The tumour displays some tubular differentiation with moderate dilatation of a few tubules. The stroma is relatively sparse.   H & E × 96

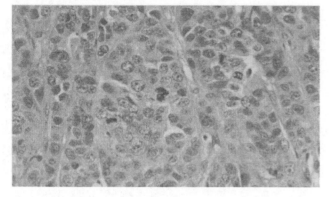

Figure 12.7 Infiltrating duct carcinoma, poorly-differentiated (Grade III). In this neoplasm there is a complete lack of tubular differentiation, the nuclei are large and pleomorphic, and there are numerous mitotic figures many of which are abnormal. H & E × 240

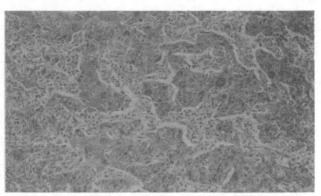

Figure 12.8 Infiltrating duct carcinoma (Grade III). This tumour is composed of irregularly shaped masses of cohesive cancer cells, displaying marked nuclear pleomorphism. Mitotic figures are numerous. The stroma is relatively scanty, being loosely fibrillary and containing some lymphocytes. The lymphoid infiltrate is insufficient for the neoplasm to be classified as a typical medullary carcinoma. H & E × 96

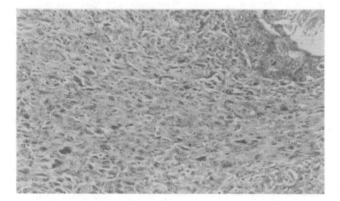

Figure 12.9 Carcinoma with undifferentiated spindle-cell (sarcomatoid) growth pattern. In the top right-hand corner of the photomicrograph there is a group of cohesive carcinoma cells: the rest of the field is occupied by loosely-arranged, pleomorphic, spheroidal, ovoid and fusiform malignant cells with a sarcomatoid growth pattern. The anaplastic cells are regarded as dedifferentiated carcinomatous elements. H & E × 96

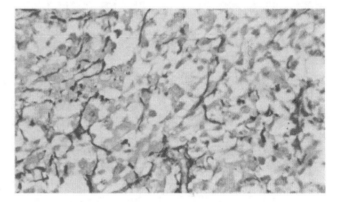

Figure 12.10 Carcinoma with sarcomatoid growth pattern. A reticulin preparation of the sarcomatoid component showing sparsity and wide separation of the fibrils; a pattern supporting the concept of the cells being carcinomatous rather than sarcomatous. Silver impregnation for reticulin × 240

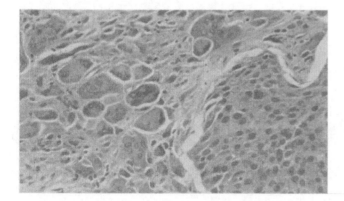

Figure 12.11 Mammary carcinoma with tumour giant cells. Section of a breast tumour from a 61-year-old woman. On the right, there is a mass of cohesive carcinoma cells. In the rest of the field, there are more loosely arranged, pleomorphic cells including many multinucleated giant forms. The large, irregular hyperchromatic nuclei of the giant cells indicate their neoplastic nature and contrast with those of the granulomatous giant cells in Figure 12.17. H & E × 240

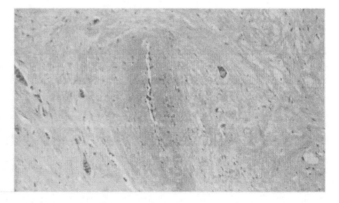

Figure 12.12 Mammary carcinoma with dense fibrotic stroma. Sections of an infiltrating duct carcinoma of the breast, showing a few widely scattered groups of cancer cells in a dense fibrous stroma. There is abundant mature collagen, but fibrocytes are small and sparse. A compressed blood vessel is present in the centre of the field. H & E × 96

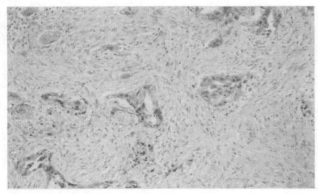

Figure 12.13 Mammary carcinoma with cellular stroma. This section shows irregularly-shaped clusters of carcinoma cells in a stroma containing numerous fibroblasts with plump nuclei.   H & E × 96

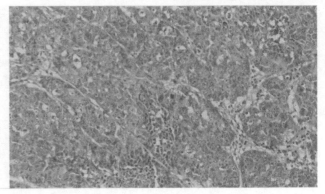

Figure 12.14 Infiltrating duct carcinoma with sparse stroma. Sections of a poorly differentiated infiltrating duct carcinoma in which the tumour is composed predominantly of irregular clumps of moderately pleomorphic malignant cells. The stroma is extremely sparse.   H & E × 96

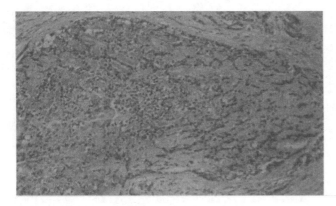

Figure 12.15 Mammary carcinoma with mucoid stroma. This section shows small, spheroidal carcinoma cells arranged as irregular cords in a stroma rich in basophilic mucin. In contrast to mucoid carcinoma, the mucin does not react positively to the periodic-acid Schiff technique, but it stains strongly with Alcian blue (see Figure 12.16).   H & E × 96

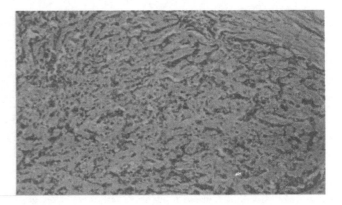

Figure 12.16 Mammary carcinoma with mucoid stroma. A further section of the tumour illustrated in Figure 12.15. The stromal mucin is stained blue.   Alcian blue × 96

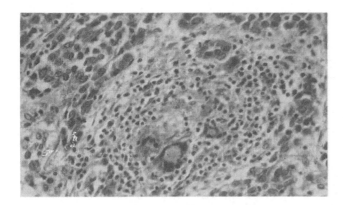

Figure 12.17 Mammary carcinoma with stromal granulomas. The centre of the field is occupied by a non-caseating granuloma composed of histiocytes, lymphocytes and multinucleated giant cells. Micro-organisms could not be demonstrated. The granuloma is surrounded by infiltrating spheroidal carcinoma cells.   H & E × 240

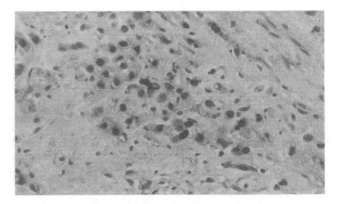

Figure 12.18 Mammary carcinoma: radiation change. A drill biopsy from a breast cancer after irradiation to a dose of 2400 rad. Many of the tumour cells have homogenized, hyperchromatic nuclei and vacuolated cytoplasm; some have undergone fusion to form syncytial clusters.   H & E × 240

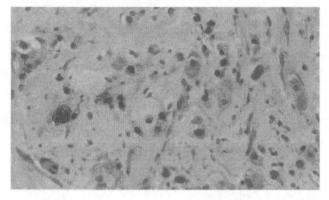

Figure 12.19 Mammary carcinoma: radiation change. Another part of the tumour illustrated in Figure 12.18. The cells have shrunk away from the oedematous stroma. The cytoplasm is vacuolated. Many of the nuclei are hyperchromatic and homogenous, while others display karyolysis. A multinucleated tumour cell is present on the left. H & E × 240

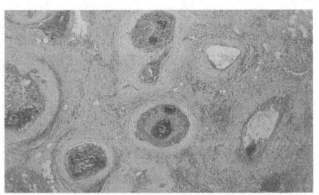

Figure 12.20 Comedo carcinoma of the breast. Section of a mammary tumour which was predominantly intraductal. In this field, the duct walls are thickened and their lumina are distended by malignant cells. Central necrosis and dystrophic calcification have occurred in many of the ducts. H & E × 24

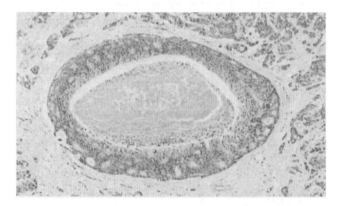

Figure 12.21 Comedo-type necrosis in metastatic mammary carcinoma. Section of an adrenal gland containing secondary carcinoma from the breast. The large ovoid mass of cancer cells, occupying most of the field, shows central coagulative necrosis and a cribriform pattern in the viable tumour of the peripheral zone, thus simulating comedo intraduct carcinoma as seen in primary breast cancer. H & E × 96

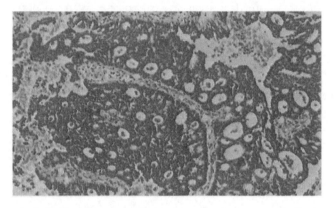

Figure 12.22 Secondary deposit of mammary carcinoma in vertebral body. This illustrates the formation of a cribriform pattern in a metastatic deposit. The primary tumour was a cribriform intraduct and infiltrating carcinoma of the breast. H & E × 96

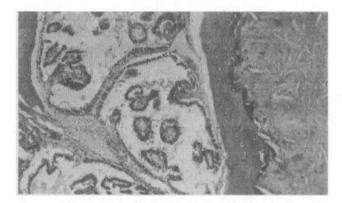

Figure 12.23 Papillary carcinoma of the breast, metastatic to bone. The patient had an intraduct and infiltrating papillary carcinoma of the breast. Eighteen months after mastectomy, she developed spinal cord compression, and secondary tumour was found in the vertebrae when laminectomy was performed. The section illustrated here was prepared from the vertebral biopsy. The papillary pattern is retained in the metastic deposit. Bone trabeculae are seen at the left and right of the field. H & E × 96

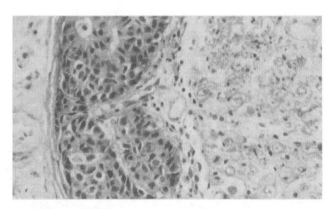

Figure 12.24 Neural invasion by mammary carcinoma. Section of part of the brachial plexus from a patient with infiltrating duct carcinoma of the breast. The right half of the field is occupied by myelinated nerve fibres cut transversely. Between this bundle of nerve fibres and the perineurium on the left, there is a mass of pleomorphic carcinoma cells. H & E × 240

clast-like giant cells are seen in the stroma of a carcinoma (see Chapter 16) and sometimes giant-cell
granulomas are present (Figure 12.17). The significance of these changes is not known. The possible
prognostic significance of elastosis within the stroma of
mammary carcinomas is discussed later, in Chapter 18.

Considerable alteration, both in the stroma and in the
neoplastic cells, may be seen after radiotherapy and
some of these changes are illustrated in Figures 12.18
and 12.19.

In situ duct carcinoma is found in association with
most, but not all, infiltrating duct carcinomas, provided
sampling is adequate. Both the proportion and pattern
of *in situ* duct carcinoma associated with infiltrating
tumours has been associated with prognosis[4].

In some classifications, infiltrating duct carcinoma
with a predominantly intraductal component and only
minimal infiltration is classified separately from predominantly infiltrating carcinoma, because the former is
associated with a more favourable prognosis than with
most infiltrating duct carcinomas. For example, some
workers consider invasive carcinoma with a predominantly comedo intraductal component (Figure
12.20) as a special type[5]. However, it must be appreciated that the invasive component of a carcinoma
occasionally shows comedo-like necrosis and this
pattern may even be seen in metastatic lesions (Figure
12.21). Clearly this must not be confused with a true *in
situ* lesion. In fact, not only a comedo pattern, but other
configurations commonly seen in intraduct carcinoma
can also be p.esent in infiltrating neoplasms and their
metastases. This applies to both cribriform and papillary
patterns (Figures 12.22 and 12.23). Usually such
patterns are not predominant within the invasive
component but occasionally they are, as in the series of
pure infiltrating papillary carcinomas reviewed by Fisher
et al. (see Chapter 16)[6], and the predominantly infiltra-

ting cribriform carcinomas recently described by Page
et al.[7]. Such tumours are associated with a relatively
good prognosis.

The invasive component of carcinoma not only infiltrates the stroma of the breast but may also be seen
within lymphatics, blood vessels and perineural spaces
(Figure 12.24). Vascular and lymphatic invasion are
illustrated, and their prognostic significance considered,
in Chapter 18.

Infiltrating duct carcinoma NOS is not infrequently
seen in combination with other specialized types of
invasive duct carcinoma and sometimes with invasive
lobular carcinoma.

References

1. Fisher, E.R., Gregorio, R.M. and Fisher, B. (1975). The
   pathology of invasive breast cancer. *Cancer*, **36**, 1–85
2. Gallager, H.S. and Martin, J.E. (1969). Early phases in the
   development of breast cancer. *Cancer*, **24**, 1170–1178
3. Bloom, H.J.G. and Richardson, W.W. (1957). Histological
   grading and prognosis in breast cancer. *Br. J. Cancer*, **11**,
   359–377
4. Silverberg, S.G. and Chitale, A.R. (1973). Assessment of significance of proportions of intraductal and infiltrating tumour
   growth in ductal carcinoma of the breast. *Cancer*, **32**, 830–837
5. McDivitt, R.W., Stewart, F.W. and Berg, J.W. (1968). Tumours
   of the breast. In *Atlas of Tumour Pathology*, 2nd Series, Fascicle
   2, p. 54. (Washington DC: Armed Forces Institute of Pathology)
6. Fisher, E.R., Palekar, A.S., Redmond, C., Barton, B. and Fisher,
   B. (1980). Pathologic findings from the National Surgical
   Adjuvant Breast Project (Protocol No. 4) VI. Invasive papillary
   cancer. *Am. J. Clin. Pathol.*, **73**, 313–321
7. Page, D.L., Dixon, J.M., Anderson, T.J., Lee, D. and Stewart,
   H.J. (1983). Invasive cribriform carcinoma of the breast. *Histopathology*, **7**, 525–536

Infiltrating Lobular Carcinoma

The reported incidence of infiltrating lobular carcinoma varies from 1 to 20%[1]; although the variation may in part be due to genuine geographical differences, it is probable that it mainly reflects the fact that some of the rarer microscopic patterns of the tumour have only recently been recognized. The true incidence is probably around 12% of all breast carcinomas. The incidence of lobular carcinoma is relatively low in Japanese women[2]. The average age of women with infiltrating lobular carcinoma is similar to that for women with infiltrating breast cancer in general and is 5–10 years greater than for women with *in situ* lobular carcinoma. As with lobular carcinoma *in situ* the incidence of bilateral carcinoma is high[3].

On gross examination infiltrating lobular carcinoma is often rubbery and less well defined than infiltrating duct carcinoma. The most widely recognized and best described histological pattern of infiltrating lobular carcinoma is shown in Figures 13.1–13.4, where the cells are disposed individually or as single files ('Indian files') in a fibroblastic stroma. Figure 13.3 illustrates the so-called 'targetoid' pattern, in which the single files of cells are arranged in concentric rings around the normal ducts. Even in the less well recognized variants of infiltrating lobular carcinoma, this single file pattern is usually present to a greater or lesser degree somewhere within the tumour. The cells of infiltrating lobular carcinoma lack cohesion and have a rather bland monomorphic appearance, being smaller and less pleomorphic than those of infiltrating duct carcinoma. This has led to occasional use of the term 'small cell carcinoma' for this type of tumour. However, as with lobular carcinoma *in situ*, the cells of invasive lobular carcinoma are sometimes slightly larger and show mild to moderate pleomorphism.

Less common patterns of infiltrating lobular carcinoma have now been recognized and have been well described by Martinez and Azzopardi[1]. Trabeculae of neoplastic cells which vary in size are seen to a limited degree in about half of all infiltrating lobular carcinomas. The loose alveolar arrangement illustrated in Figures 13.5 and 13.6 is another recently recognized pattern and is seen relatively frequently, but the alveolar arrangement composed of cohesive cells illustrated in Figure 13.7 is rather less common. An alveolar pattern is sometimes seen at the infiltrating margin of a tumour which shows another pattern of infiltration in the more central area. It is occasionally difficult to distinguish an infiltrating tumour with an alveolar arrangement from *in situ* lobular carcinoma with massive distension of the acini (Figure 13.8). Solid variants of infiltrating lobular carcinoma also occur (Figures 13.9–13.12). Fechner[4] described a pattern composed of confluent sheets of cells arranged in irregularly-shaped solid nests. Martinez and Azzopardi[1] illustrated aggregates of dissociated cells which they distinguished from the solid pattern of Fechner[4]. Van Bogaert and Maldague[5] also recognized a confluent solid pattern of infiltrating lobular carcinoma. In the past, tubular carcinoma has always been considered to be a type of infiltrating duct carcinoma, but recently it has been recognized that some carcinomas with a tubular pattern are variants of infiltrating lobular carcinoma[6]. The tubules are usually small and many have indistinct lumina (Figure 13.13).

Intracytoplasmic droplets of mucin, similar to those seen in lobular carcinoma *in situ*, are present in about 25% of the cells in most cases of infiltrating lobular carcinoma[7]. However, this pattern of mucin secretion is not exclusive to lobular carcinoma and may be seen in other forms of mammary carcinoma, albeit less frequently[5]. The characteristic appearance of the intracytoplasmic droplets can occasionally prove helpful in predicting the site of an occult primary carcinoma in the case of metastatic disease (Figure 13.14). Granular mucin is less common in lobular carcinoma. Foci of true signet-ring cells can also occur (Figure 13.15), but tumours composed predominantly of signet-ring cells are best regarded as a separate tumour type.

The amount and nature of the stroma also varies considerably. In some lobular carcinomas fibrous stroma is extensive, whilst in others there is little or no productive fibrosis. The old term 'scirrhous carcinoma' undoubtedly included some infiltrating lobular carcinomas. Tumours with little or no productive fibrosis may be very hard to detect on gross examination and on mammography, as there may be minimal change in density between the tumour and surrounding normal breast tissue. In some tumours the malignant cells are so sparsely distributed within very abundant stroma that they are easily overlooked on microscopic examination. Another feature characteristic of lobular carcinoma is the frequent occurrence of separate foci of infiltration, with intervening areas of normal breast tissue sometimes known as 'skip' areas.

Differentiation between invasive duct and invasive lobular carcinoma is not always easy and in a considerable proportion of cases the two cannot be distinguished. Differentiation depends on the overall structural and cytological appearance rather than on any one specific criterion (Figures 13.16 and 13.17), and it must be appreciated that combined lobular and duct carcinomas also occur. *In situ* lobular carcinoma is present in association with over 50% of cases of infiltrating lobular carcinoma but its presence is not essential to the diagnosis[8] and, indeed, occasionally *in situ* duct carcinoma may be seen adjacent to an infiltrating lobular carcinoma.

Lymph node metastases from infiltrating lobular carcinoma frequently have a characteristic pattern of infiltration (see Chapter 19) often involving the sinu-

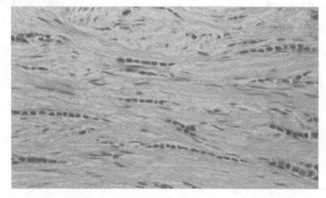

Figure 13.1 Infiltrating lobular carcinoma. Section showing a single-file ('Indian-file') pattern of infiltration, with thin columns of small, hyperchromatic tumour cells dispersed in an abundant fibroblastic stroma.   H & E × 240

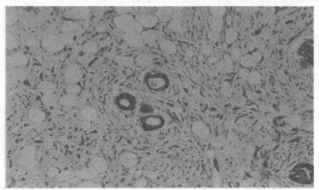

Figure 13.2 Infiltrating lobular carcinoma. Dissociated cell pattern, with individual carcinoma cells scattered in a fibrous stroma, invading the adipose tissue and infiltrating around the mammary ducts.   H & E × 96

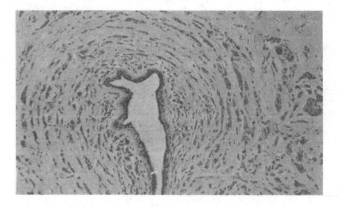

Figure 13.3 Infiltrating lobular carcinoma. An example of the targetoid pattern, in which thin columns of infiltrating tumour cells form concentric rings around a central duct. Occasional trabeculae of cells two or three layers thick are also present.   H & E × 96

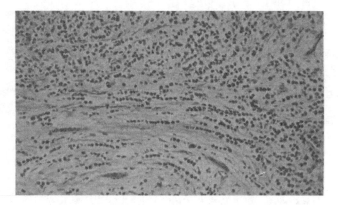

Figure 13.4 Infiltrating lobular carcinoma. The tumour comprises small, darkly-staining carcinoma cells, disposed singly and in narrow columns in a fibroblastic stroma.   H & E × 96

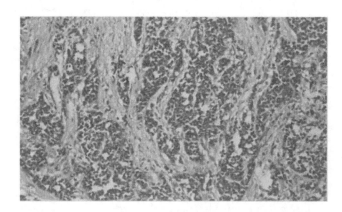

Figure 13.5 Infiltrating lobular carcinoma. In this tumour the neoplastic cells are loosely arranged in an irregular alveolar grouping with a fibroblastic stroma, in contrast to the more conventional single-file ('Indian-file') and targetoid configurations.   H & E × 96

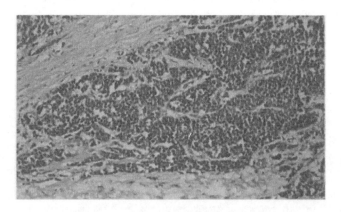

Figure 13.6 Infiltrating lobular carcinoma. Another example of loose, alveolar grouping of the tumour cells in a fibrous stroma.   H & E × 96

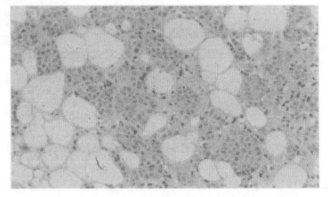

Figure 13.7 Infiltrating lobular carcinoma. In this tumour the malignant cells form cohesive masses, producing a solid alveolar growth pattern in contrast to the loose alveolar pattern illustrated in Figures 13.5 and 13.6, and to the more conventional patterns illustrated previously.   H & E × 96

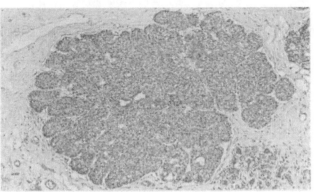

Figure 13.8 Lobular carcinoma *in situ*. In this lesion the acini have become markedly expanded by the proliferating neoplastic cells, and are closely apposed so that the intervening stroma is relatively inconspicuous. This might be confused with the solid alveolar type of infiltrating lobular carcinoma shown in Figure 13.7. Nevertheless, the general architectural configuration of the lobule is retained, and there has been no penetration of the basement membranes.   H & E × 96

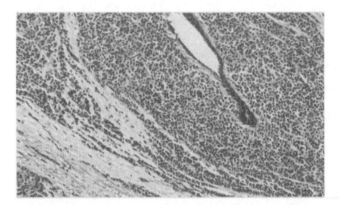

Figure 13.9 Infiltrating lobular carcinoma. In this section there is prominent cuffing of a duct by a broad mass of carcinoma cells. The cells are loosely arranged and generally lack cohesion but do not show the wide dispersion seen in the classical targetoid pattern.   H & E × 96

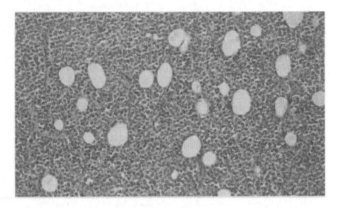

Figure 13.10 Infiltrating lobular carcinoma. Diffuse infiltration of mammary adipose tissue with wide separation of the fat cells: a pattern of invasion reminiscent of a malignant lymphoma. The demonstration of mucin in the cytoplasm of many of the tumour cells confirmed the diagnosis of carcinoma.   H & E × 96

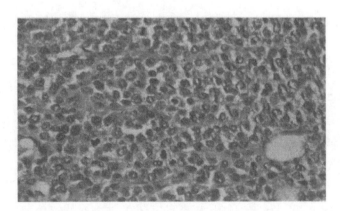

Figure 13.11 Infiltrating lobular carcinoma. A higher magnification of the neoplasm illustrated in Figure 13.10. This lobular carcinoma is of the large-cell type. The cells are spheroidal and display many mitotic figures.   H & E × 240

Figure 13.12 Infiltrating lobular carcinoma. In this tumour, the cancer cells are disposed as large, solid masses in which cellular cohesion is more marked.   H & E × 96

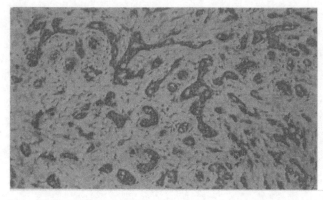

Figure 13.13 Infiltrating lobular carcinoma. An invasive tumour of lobular type with tubular differentiation. The tubules are small, often with indistinct lumina, and the stroma is myxoid.   H & E × 96

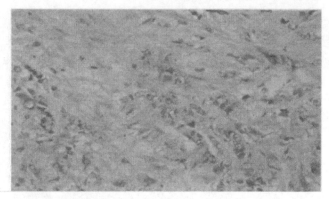

Figure 13.14 Lobular carcinoma of breast, metastatic to small intestine. The patient presented with abdominal symptoms. Laparotomy was performed, a length of small intestine resected, and a histological diagnosis of malignant lymphoma returned. However, the application of special stains revealed mucin droplets in many of the tumour cells, and a revised diagnosis of secondary carcinoma was suggested. Further investigations finally established the diagnosis of disseminated lobular carcinoma of the breast. This section was prepared from the wall of the small intestine. It shows infiltration by spheroidal carcinoma cells, most of which contain mucin droplets, stained red.   PAS after diastase digestion × 240

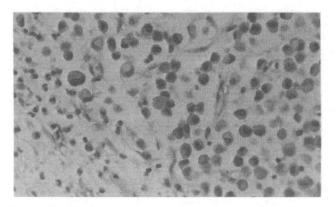

Figure 13.15 Infiltrating lobular carcinoma. This tumour contained foci of signet-ring cells as illustrated here. Although signet-ring cells may occur in lobular carcinoma, tumours composed predominantly of such cells are usually classified as a separate type (signet-ring cell carcinoma).   H & E × 240

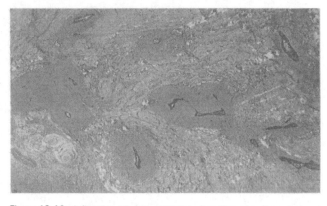

Figure 13.16 Infiltrating lobular carcinoma. A section showing prominent periductal elastosis, appearing as brightly-eosinophilic cuffs around the ducts. The intervening stroma is infiltrated by narrow columns and small clusters of carcinoma cells. Such marked elastosis is more commonly seen with infiltrating duct carcinoma. In the tumour illustrated here, the cytology, the invasion pattern and the presence of *in situ* neoplasia in the lobules all indicated a lobular carcinoma.   H & E × 24

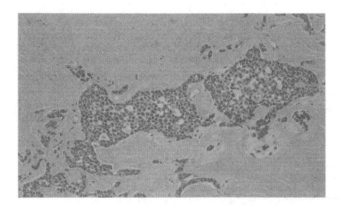

Figure 13.17 Infiltrating lobular carcinoma. A pattern in which the abundance and density of the fibrous stroma is more reminiscent of an infiltrating duct carcinoma of 'scirrhous' type. However, the cell type was judged to be lobular, and lobular carcinoma *in situ* was present in the adjacent breast. H & E × 96

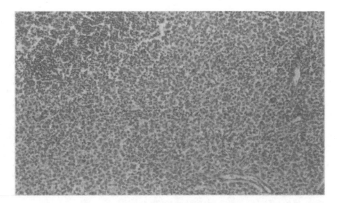

Figure 13.18 Axillary lymph node: secondary lobular carcinoma of the breast. Residual lymphocytes are present in the top left-hand corner of the field. The tumour cells are loosely arranged and generally lack cohesion; they are quite regular in size and shape in contrast to the pleomorphism usually seen in duct carcinoma. There is a striking lack of stromal reaction. A secondary neoplasm with this pattern must be distinguished from a malignant lymphoma.   H & E × 96

soids[3,5] or replacing the entire node when differentiation from a lymphoma may be difficult (Figure 13.18).

There is considerable disagreement in the literature concerning the prognosis associated with invasive lobular carcinoma; some claim that patients with this type of tumour do better than those with infiltrating duct carcinoma NOS, and others that they fare worse. In the past, little attempt has been made to relate prognosis to the different histological patterns of infiltration, but in a recent report Dixon *et al.*[9] studied the prognostic significance of four different histological patterns. They found that patients with tumours showing the classical single file and targetoid patterns had a relatively good prognosis. Patients with the alveolar variant also did comparatively well. In contrast, those with tumours showing the solid pattern of infiltration or tumours with a mixed pattern did badly.

References

1. Martinez, V. and Azzopardi, J. G. (1979). Invasive lobular carcinoma of the breast: incidence and variants. *Histopathology*, **3**, 467–488

2. Rosen, P. P., Ashikari, R., Thaler, H., Ishikawa, S., Hirota, T., Abe, O., Yamamoto, H., Beattie, E. J. Jr., Urban, J. A. and Mike, V. (1977). A comparative study of some pathologic features of mammary carcinoma in Tokyo, Japan and New York, U.S.A. *Cancer*, **39**, 429–434

3. Wheeler, J. E. and Enterline, H. T. (1976). Lobular carcinoma of the breast *in situ* and infiltrating. In Sommers, S. C. (ed.) *Pathology Annual*, **11**, pp. 161–188. (New York: Appleton-Century-Crofts)

4. Fechner, R. E. (1975). Histologic variants of infiltrating lobular carcinoma of the breast. *Hum. Pathol.*, **6**, 373–378

5. van Bogaert, L.-J. and Maldague, P. (1980). Infiltrating lobular carcinoma of the female breast. *Cancer*, **45**, 979–984

6. Fisher, E. R., Gregorio, R. M., Redmond, C. and Fisher, B. (1977). Tubulolobular invasive breast cancer: a variant of lobular invasive cancer. *Hum. Pathol.*, **8**, 679–683

7 Gad, A. and Azzopardi, J. G. (1975). Lobular carcinoma of the breast: a special variant of mucin-secreting carcinoma. *J. Clin. Pathol.*, **28**, 711–716

8. Fechner, R. E. (1972). Infiltrating lobular carcinoma without lobular carcinoma *in situ*. *Cancer*, **29**, 1539–1545

9. Dixon, J. M., Anderson, T. J., Page, D. L., Lee, D. and Duffy, S. W. (1982). Infiltrating lobular carcinoma of the breast. *Histopathology*, **6**, 149–161

Medullary Carcinoma with Lymphoid Stroma

This special type of mammary carcinoma is usually considered to be a variant of infiltrating duct carcinoma. Medullary carcinoma with lymphoid stroma is of particular interest as it is generally found to be associated with a better prognosis than the more common variants of infiltrating duct carcinoma, despite cytological features which would suggest an aggressive pattern of behaviour, and even when lymph node metastases are present[1-3]. However, this contention has been challenged by some authorities[4,5]. When the tumour does prove fatal death usually occurs within 5 years of diagnosis[3]. There has been some disparity in the literature regarding the age distribution of medullary carcinoma. Ridolfi and colleagues[3] found only a third of patients with typical medullary carcinoma to be premenopausal as compared with a half of those with non-medullary carcinoma. Neither did they find an increased familial incidence of breast cancer amongst their patients with medullary carcinoma nor in the whole group was there an increase of bilaterality. In the past, both these features have been claimed to be characteristic of medullary carcinoma. However, more recently Rosen et al.[6] have reported a significantly lower mean age incidence in patients with medullary carcinoma. Rosen and colleagues[7] also found a strong correlation with maternal breast carcinoma but a low incidence of carcinoma amongst the patients' sisters. In several comparative studies the incidence of medullary carcinoma has been found to be relatively high in Japanese women[8].

Macroscopically, medullary carcinomas are characterized by their sharp demarcation, rounded outline and soft consistency, an appearance which can give rise to an erroneous diagnosis of a benign lesion on both gross and mammographic examination (Figure 14.1). Early descriptions of medullary carcinomas emphasize their large size[1]. However, in more recent reviews the average size of medullary carcinoma has been found to be no greater than that for non-medullary tumours[3].

The typical microscopic appearance of the tumour is shown in Figures 14.2–14.7. Anastamosing syncytial sheets of malignant cells are surrounded by stroma containing large numbers of lymphocytes and plasmacytes. Sometimes lymphocytic aggregates with reaction centres are present. The malignant cells are large and markedly pleomorphic, with prominent nucleoli and numerous mitotic figures; foci of necrosis are frequent. The sheets of large pleomorphic cells may be surrounded by smaller, more elongated, cells with denser cytoplasm[9]. Squamous metaplasia is also relatively common in this type of tumour (Figure 14.6). Mucin production is inconspicuous and calcification has not been described. The characteristic well-circumscribed outline of the tumour is shown in Figure 14.7.

The increased survival rate associated with this type of carcinoma is greatest in patients with typical medullary carcinoma as illustrated in the photomicrographs. Tumours displaying some but not all of the characteristic features have been termed 'atypical medullary carcinomas'[3]. In such tumours the predominant growth pattern (75% or more) is still syncytial, but any two of the following atypical features may be present: focal tumour infiltration at the margins, mild or negligible lymphoid infiltrate, a lymphoid infiltrate confined to the periphery of the growth, nuclei with few mitoses and little pleomorphism, the presence of glandular orientation and associated intraduct carcinoma. The prognosis with this type of tumour lies between that of typical medullary carcinoma and conventional infiltrating duct carcinoma. However, the presence of intraduct carcinoma at the periphery of an otherwise typical medullary carcinoma does not appear to influence the prognosis. On the other hand, tumours in the atypical group with a sparse lymphoid infiltrate are associated with a relatively poor prognosis. Tumours with a syncytial growth pattern comprising less than 75% of the whole tumour or those with three or more atypical features were considered non-medullary infiltrating duct carcinomas by Ridolfi et al.[3]. When strict diagnostic criteria are applied, typical medullary carcinoma accounts for only about 3% of all infiltrating mammary carcinomas.

Mucoid Carcinoma (Colloid, Gelatinous, Mucinous or Mucin-producing Carcinoma).

Pure mucoid carcinomas account for about 2% of all mammary carcinomas. They are associated with a better prognosis than most infiltrating duct carcinomas but this improved outlook applies only to those tumours which are uniformly mucoid, and not to infiltrating tumours with only a partial mucoid pattern[10-12]. Furthermore, a recent report by Rosen[13] indicates that the mortality rate even for pure mucoid carcinomas is not so favourable on long term follow-up.

There is disagreement in the literature as to whether or not mucoid carcinomas occur more often in older age groups[10-12]. On average, mucoid carcinomas tend to be slightly larger than conventional infiltrating duct carcinomas[10-12]. On macroscopic examination, the tumours have a typical gelatinous appearance (Figure 14.8). On microscopic examination, groups of malignant cells, usually showing little pleomorphism and a low mitotic rate, appear to float in pools of mucin surrounded by bands of fibrous connective tissue (Figure 14.9, 14.10). The large amount of extracellular mucin which is the characteristic feature of these tumours is sometimes difficult to visualize in sections stained with haematoxylin and eosin, but is well demonstrated by staining with the Alcian blue or PAS techniques (Figure 14.11). Sometimes focal areas of calcification occur within the

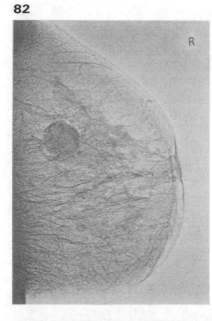

Figure 14.1 Medullary carcinoma: xeromammogram. A xeromammogram showing the neoplasm as a sharply-defined rounded density which could easily be mistaken for a benign lesion

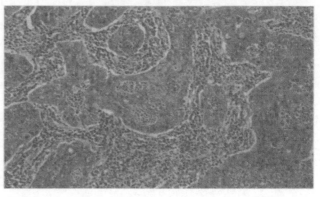

Figure 14.2 Medullary carcinoma with lymphoid stroma. The neoplasm is composed of clusters and trabeculae of large polyhedral cells. The stroma is infiltrated with many lymphocytes and plasmacytes, some of which are also present within the tumour cell masses. H & E × 96

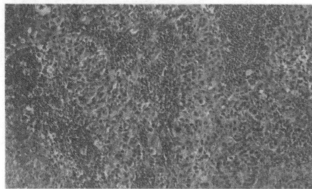

Figure 14.3 Medullary carcinoma with lymphoid stroma. Macroscopically the tumour was a sharply-defined soft, greyish, spheroidal mass, 2 cm in diameter. In this section the epithelial cell masses are much less clearly defined than in Figure 14.2 as a result of encroachment by the lymphoid infiltrate. Here there are irregular trabeculae of large, pleomorphic carcinoma cells, displaying many mitotic figures. The intervening stroma contains numerous darkly-staining lymphoid cells. H & E × 96

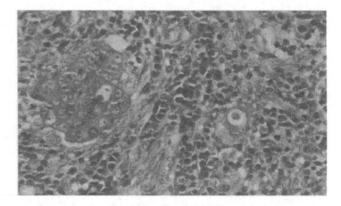

Figure 14.4 Medullary carcinoma with lymphoid stroma. A clump of tumour cells, with vesicular nuclei and quite prominent nucleoli, is present on the left. This section illustrates the large number of plasmacytes which are often found in the lymphoid infiltrate; their cytoplasm is stained deep red in this Unna–Pappenheim preparation. Methyl green/pyronin × 240

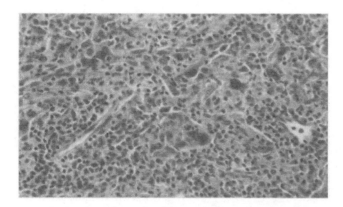

Figure 14.5 Medullary carcinoma with lymphoid stroma. The carcinoma cells display marked nuclear pleomorphism with some giant forms. They are largely disassociated by the abundant lymphocytic and plasmacytic infiltrate. H & E × 240

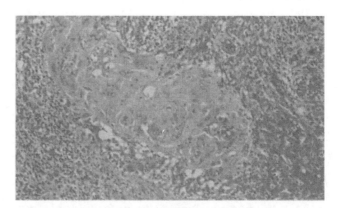

Figure 14.6 Medullary carcinoma: squamous metaplasia. Section of a breast tumour which had all the features of a typical medullary carcinoma, and additionally displayed patchy squamous metaplasia. This photograph shows a large group of carcinoma cells which have abundant eosinophilic cytoplasm. Although there is no keratinization, prickle-cells were clearly demonstrable microscopically. H & E × 96

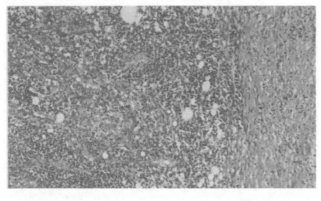

Figure 14.7 Medullary carcinoma with lymphoid stroma. Section illustrating the sharp peripheral circumscription of tumours of this type. The neoplasm consists of large spheroidal cells intermingled with numerous lymphocytes and plasmacytes.   H & E × 96

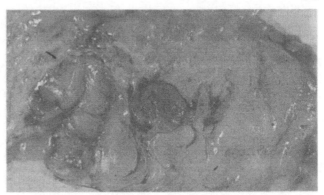

Figure 14.8 Mucoid carcinoma of the breast. The cut surface of a bisected surgical specimen, showing a sharply-defined, spheroidal, glistening, grey, mucoid tumour in predominantly fatty breast tissue

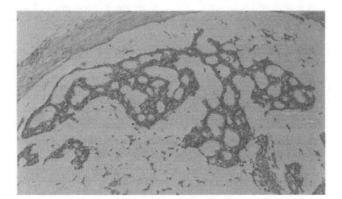

Figure 14.9 Mucoid carcinoma with trabecular (ribbon) pattern. A section showing the typical features of a mucoid carcinoma: tumour cells apparently floating in a large pool of extracellular mucin. The cells are arranged as inter-connecting trabeculae.   H & E × 96

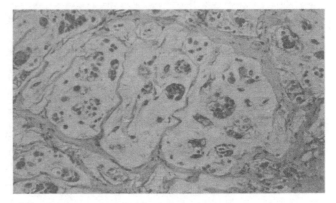

Figure 14.10 Mucoid carcinoma. Section showing the typical microscopic pattern of small clusters of carcinoma cells apparently floating in large pools of extracellular mucin. The mucin stains pale blue with the haematoxylin, and the pools are separated by thin connective tissue septa.   H & E × 96

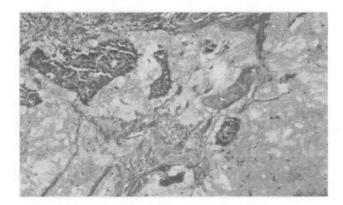

Figure 14.11 Mucoid carcinoma. In this preparation the abundant extra-cellular mucin is stained deep blue, the tumour-cell clumps mauve and the connective tissue red.   Alcian blue/neutral red × 240

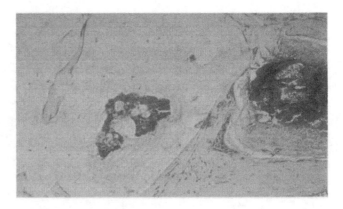

Figure 14.12 Mucoid carcinoma: focal calcification. A darkly-stained spheroidal focus of calcification is present on the extreme right. In the left half of the field, there is an irregularly shaped cluster of tumour cells in a large pool of extracellular mucin.   H & E × 96

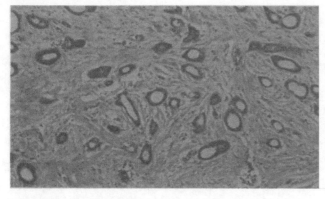

Figure 14.13 Tubular carcinoma. Section of a mammary tumour 1 cm in diameter. The carcinoma comprises irregularly-disposed, highly-differentiated, open tubules growing in an abundant fibroblastic stroma. Myoepithelial mantles are completely absent, and special stains showed basement membranes to be lacking.   H & E × 96

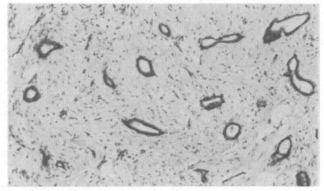

Figure 14.14   Tubular carcinoma of the breast. The carcinoma is composed of small well-formed epithelial tubules, supported by a loose-textured, moderately cellular fibrous stroma. The tubules lack both basement membranes and myoepithelial mantles.   H & E × 96

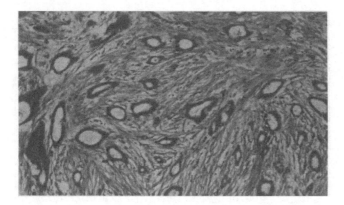

Figure 14.15   Tubular carcinoma of the breast. The tubules of benign proliferative lesions of the breast are usually surrounded by basement membranes which can be demonstrated by the PAS or trichrome techniques. Basement membranes are absent from around the tubules of a carcinoma. In the section illustrated here, collagen is stained blue. Basement membranes would appear as thin blue-stained rings around the tubules: however, such structures are absent, and the arrangement of the tubules in relation to the stromal collagen fibres is irregular and haphazard.   Picro–Mallory × 96

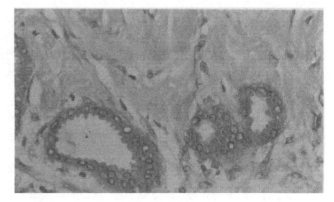

Figure 14.16   Tubular carcinoma. Section showing a group of three tubules illustrating the intraluminal cytoplasmic projections (snouts) protruding from the luminal surfaces of the tumour cells and the lack of myoepithelial layers.   H & E × 240

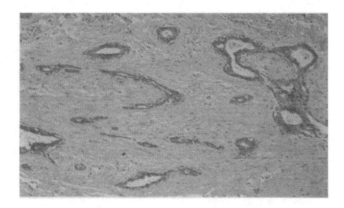

Figure 14.17   Sclerosing adenosis: for comparison with Figures 14.13–14.15. The fibrous stroma is denser than that of the tubular carcinoma. The tubules are irregular in size and shape and, although the myoepithelium is attenuated in places, a double cell layer is apparent around most of the ducts.   H & E × 96

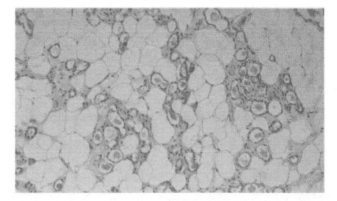

Figure 14.18   Microglandular adenosis: for comparison with Figures 14.13–14.15. The tubules are small, rounded and regular, and contain eosinophilic material. They lie within adipose tissue and there is no fibroblastic stromal response. The tubules are lined by a single layer of regular cuboidal cells with no evidence of intraluminal cytoplasmic projections. In microglandular adenosis myoepithelial cells are not usually detectable.   H & E × 96

mucoid pools (Figure 14.12). Although small amounts of intracellular mucin may be present, tumours in which intracytoplasmic mucin predominates (signet-ring cell carcinomas) are deemed to comprise a separate group. *In situ* duct carcinoma is occasionally found in association with mucoid carcinomas, and sometimes the intraductal component contains a large amount of extracellular mucin.

Recent studies have suggested that some mucoid carcinomas of the breast are related to carcinoid tumours, since cytoplasmic argyrophilia has been demonstrated and neurosecretory granules have been found on electron microscopic examination[14,15]. Capella and colleagues[15] divide mucoid carcinomas into two groups, designated A and B. Type A tumours have abundant extracellular mucin, but sparse intracellular mucin. The cells are arranged in ribbons or rings (Figure 14.9) and usually display hyaline cytoplasm, hyperchromatic nuclei, and some pleomorphism; they are not argyrophilic. Type B tumours also have abundant extracellular mucin, but intracellular mucin is more plentiful than in type A. The malignant cells are arranged in clumps (Figure 14.10), their cytoplasm is granular, and the nuclei are more uniform; it is in this group that argyrophilia is usually demonstrable. The incidence of type A and type B tumours is about equal and combined type A and B tumours also occur. Capella *et al.*[15] found a striking difference in mean age between their two groups of mucoid carcinomas – 61.4 years for type A tumours and 75 years for type B tumours.

Although mucoid carcinoma is usually considered a variant of duct carcinoma, a few may be variants of lobular carcinoma. Mixed tumours with the appearance of both mucoid carcinoma and features more typical of carcinoid tumours also occur.

Tubular or Well-differentiated Carcinoma

Tubular carcinoma has recently been delineated as a specific type of mammary tumour, because of its characteristic microscopic appearance, low metastatic potential and relatively favourable prognosis[16-20]. The reported incidence varies from about 0.5 to 10% of all mammary carcinomas[17-19]. This wide range may be due in part to the different criteria used to delineate these tumours[18]. The incidence of tubular carcinoma found in most screening clinics is relatively high[16], probably due to two factors: (1) the tumours, although small and therefore often impalpable, have a very irregular outline easily recognizable on mammography and (2) calcification is often present.

The mean age of patients with tubular carcinoma has been found to be slightly lower than that for patients with other forms of mammary carcinoma[17-20]. One recent study reported a significant association with a family history of breast carcinoma[17]. Several studies have shown an increased incidence of multicentricity in patients with tubular carcinoma, and some also an association with bilaterality[17]. Tubular carcinoma has also been described in the male breast[21].

The tumours are usually small, the majority being less than 2 cm in maximum diameter, and have a stellate outline. The histological appearances are illustrated in Figures 14.13–14.16. Small, irregular tubular stuctures are surrounded by abundant stroma which is usually cellular but may be collagenous or even hyalinized. Prominent elastosis is often present. The tubules are open, many have angulated contours and they are lined by single layers of rather uniform neoplastic cells

showing little atypia and very few mitotic figures. Occasional trabecular bars may be present within the tubules but branching and anastomosis of the tubules is not a feature. The cytoplasm is characteristically pale and frequently apical snouts project into the lumina (Figure 14.16). Differentiation from sclerosing adenosis, especially when radial scars are present, can be difficult.

Examination of both the epithelial and stromal elements is helpful in distinguishing sclerosing adenosis, including radial scars, from carcinoma. Both myoepithelial mantles and PAS-positive basement membrane material can usually be demonstrated around benign tubules, although either may be indistinct or defective around individual tubules. In contrast infiltrating carcinoma features neither *pari passu* proliferation of myoepithelial cells nor regular basement membranes[22]. The stroma of sclerosing adenosis is characteristically dense, hyaline and sparsely cellular and compresses the tubular structures with frequent loss of lumina (Figure 14.17). In contrast, the stroma of tubular carcinomas is usually more loose and cellular and the lumina of the epithelial components are open. Particular attention should also be paid to the microanatomy of the lesions. In classical sclerosing adenosis, a whorled lobular pattern is still apparent and the edge of the lesion is sharply defined. Radial scars have a sclerotic centre and peripheral dilatation of the ducts, producing the 'flower-head' appearance. Carcinomas have an infiltrating edge; the centre may or may not be sclerotic.

Another common variant of adenosis, termed microglandular adenosis, may be even more difficult to distinguish from tubular carcinoma[19,23,24]. The glandular structures in microglandular adenosis, like tubular carcinoma, are lined by a single layer of cells. The myoepithelial layer, usually so helpful in distinguishing benign lesions from carcinoma, is inconspicuous or absent in microglandular adenosis. The lining cells are cuboidal or flattened without apical snouts and the cytoplasm is clear or eosinophilic. The tubules are rounded and uniform and contain eosinophilic material. They show no angulation, and trabecular bars, occasionally seen in tubular carcinoma, are absent (Figure 14.18). Peritubular basement membranes cannot be demonstrated by the PAS technique in most cases of microglandular adenosis, but silver impregnation consistently reveals complete reticulin rings around the tubules[23]. In microglandular adenosis the tubules are irregularly dispersed in adipose tissue, or within a fibrous stroma which is usually dense and often hyalinized, whereas tubular carcinoma frequently has a much more cellular stroma. Furthermore, microglandular adenosis does not have the overall infiltrating outline typical of tubular carcinoma. However, as with all benign breast lesions the possibility of coexistence of a benign and a malignant condition should always be carefully considered. Rosen[24] observed such an association in some of his cases of microglandular adenosis.

In situ duct carcinoma may be present around the edge of a tubular carcinoma and would be a further point in favour of malignancy in a controversial diagnosis The *in situ* component when present usually has a micropapillary or cribriform pattern[19]. Although not as common as *in situ* duct carcinoma, the coexistence of lobular carcinoma *in situ* with tubular carcinoma has also been described. Tubular carcinoma is considered by most authorities to be a variant of infiltrating duct carcinoma, but it has been suggested that it may be a type of infiltrating lobular carcinoma[20].

The pattern of tubular carcinoma is frequently seen in combination with more conventional infiltrating duct or lobular carcinomas, or in multicentric association with other carcinomas. The term 'tubular carcinoma' should be reserved for those tumours in which the invasive component is composed entirely of the characteristic pattern described above. The importance of distinguishing tubular carcinoma from well-differentiated infiltrating duct carcinoma NOS has also been emphasized[18,19]. It may be that tubular carcinoma represents an early phase of infiltrating duct carcinoma[19].

References

1. Moore, O. S. Jr. and Foote, F. W. Jr. (1949). The relatively favorable prognosis of medullary carcinoma of the breast. *Cancer*, **2**, 635

2. Richardson, W. W. (1956). Medullary carcinoma of the breast: a distinctive tumour type with a relatively good prognosis following radical mastectomy. *Br. J. Cancer*, **10**, 415

3. Ridolfi, R. L., Rosen, P. P., Port, A., Kinne, D. and Mike, V. (1977). Medullary carcinoma of the breast. *Cancer*, **40**, 1365

4. Flores, L., Arlen, M., Elguezabal, A. Livingston, S. F. and Levowitz, B. S. (1974). Host tumour relationships in medullary carcinoma of the breast. *Surg. Gynecol. Obstet.*, **139**, 683

5. Fisher, E. R., Redmond, C. and Fisher, B. (1980). Pathologic findings from the national surgical adjuvant breast project. (Protocol no. 4) VI. Discriminants for five-year treatment failure. *Cancer*, **46**, 908

6. Rosen, P. P., Lesser, M. L., Senie, R. T. and Duthie, K. (1982). Epidemiology of breast carcinoma IV: age and histologic tumour type. *J. Surg. Oncol.*, **19**, 44

7. Rosen, P. P., Lesser, M. L. Senie, R. T. and Kinne, D. W. (1982). Epidemiology of breast carcinoma III. Relationship of family history to tumour type. *Cancer*, **50**, 171

8. Rosen, P. P., Ashikari, R., Thaler, H., Ishikawa, S., Hirota, T., Abe, O., Yamamoto, H., Beattie, E. J. Jr., Urban, J. A. and Mike, V. (1977). A comparative study of some pathologic features of mammary carcinoma in Tokyo, Japan and New York, U.S.A. *Cancer*, **39**, 429

9. Azzopardi, J. G. (1979). *Problems in Breast Pathology*, p. 286. (Vol. 11 in Bennington, J. L. (consulting ed.) *Major Problems in Pathology*. (London, Philadelphia and Toronto: Saunders)

10. Norris, H. J. and Taylor, H. B. (1965). Prognosis of mucinous (gelatinous) carcinoma of the breast. *Cancer*, **18**, 879

11. Silverberg, S. G., Kay, S., Chitale, A. R. and Levitt, S. H. (1971). Colloid carcinoma of the breast. *Am. J. Clin. Pathol.*, **55**, 355

12. McDivitt, R. W., Stewart, F. W. and Berg, J. W. (1968). Tumours of the breast. In *Atlas of Tumour Pathology*, 2nd series, fascicle 2, p. 55. (Washington DC: Armed Forces Institute of Pathology)

13. Rosen, P. P. (1980). Colloid carcinoma of the breast: analysis of 64 patients with long-term follow-up. *Am. J. Clin. Pathol.*, **73**, 304

14. Fisher, E. R., Palekar, A. S. *et al.* (1979). Solid and mucinous varieties of so-called mammary carcinoid tumours. *Am. J. Clin. Pathol.*, **72**, 909

15. Capella, C., Eusebi, V., Mann, B. and Azzopardi, J. G. (1980). Endocrine differentiation in mucoid carcinoma of the breast. *Histopathology*, **4**, 613

16. Feig, S. A., Shaber, G. S., Patchefsky, A. S., Schwartz, G. F., Edeiken, J. and Nerlinger, R. (1978). Tubular carcinoma of the breast. *Radiology*, **129**, 311

17. Lagios, M. D., Rose, M. R. and Margolin, F. R. (1980). Tubular carcinoma of the breast. Association with multicentricity, bilaterality and family history of mammary carcinoma. *Am. J. Clin. Pathol.*, **73**, 25

18. van Bogaert, L.-J. (1982). Clinicopathologic hallmarks of mammary tubular carcinoma. *Hum. Pathol.*, **13**, 558

19. McDivitt, R. W., Boyce, W. and Gersell, D. (1982). Tubular carcinoma of the breast. Clinical and pathological observations concerning 135 cases. *Am. J. Surg. Pathol.*, **6**, 401

20. Eusebi, V., Betts, C. M. and Bussolati, G. (1979). Tubular carcinoma: a variant of secretory breast carcinoma. *Histopathology*, **3**, 407

21. Taxy, J. B. (1975). Tubular carcinoma of the male breast. *Cancer*, **36**, 462

22. Flotte, T. J., Bell, D. A. and Greco, M. A. (1980). Tubular carcinoma and sclerosing adenosis. The use of basal lamina as a differential feature. *Am. J. Surg. Pathol.*, **4**, 75

23. Clement, P. B. and Azzopardi, J. G. (1983). Microglandular adenosis of the breast – a lesion simulating tubular carcinoma. *Histopathology*, **7**, 169

24. Rosen, P. P. (1983). Microglandular adenosis. A benign lesion simulating invasive mammary carcinoma. *Am. J. Surg. Pathol.* **7**, 137

Special Types of Mammary Carcinoma 2

Carcinoid Tumour of the Breast

Both primary and secondary carcinoid tumours of the breast have been described. There has been considerable interest in primary carcinoid tumours since the description by Cubilla and Woodruff[1] of ten cases (including two in the addendum) in 1977. In their series, the patients were all female, with a mean age of 54 years. Four of the ten patients had died with widespread metastatic tumour and a fifth was alive with disseminated disease. All the patients with tumours less than 2 cm in diameter were alive. Other reports of primary carcinoid tumours of the breast have subsequently appeared in the literature, including one in a male who had bilateral mammary neoplasms and an increased urinary excretion of norepinephrine[2]. The tumours are usually well circumscribed. On histological examination they are composed of solid nests of cells with poorly defined outlines and a low mitotic rate, set within a very vascular stroma (Figure 15.1). Ribbon-like and glandular patterns also occur (Figures 15.2 and 15.3). Sometimes the cells show marked pleomorphism (Figure 15.4). Argyrophil granules can be demonstrated by a modified Grimelius technique as shown in Figures 15.5 and 15.6, but argentaffin granules are usually absent. Neurosecretory granules can be indentified on electron microscopy in some cases.

Most workers consider these tumours to be related to lobular carcinoma, but *in situ* duct carcinoma has also been identified around the margins of some mammary carcinoids. Dissension as to the true carcinoid nature of these tumours has been voiced[3,4]. The failure to correlate argyrophilia with the presence of neurosecretory granules in some cases, the absence of argyrophilia in other mammary tumours with histological similarity to carcinoid tumours and the demonstration of focal argyrophilia in examples of otherwise conventional forms of invasive breast cancer have all thrown doubt on the validity of the concept. Furthermore, in a recent study Clayton *et al.*[5] found that some of the ultrastructural dense core granules in the tumours they studied contained milk protein and not neuroendocrine polypeptides.

Recently argyrophilic granules have been identified in certain mucoid carcinomas of the breast and it has been suggested that mucoid carcinomas consist of two types, those which are related to carcinoid tumours and those which are not (see Chapter 14).

Signet-ring Cell Carcinoma

Pure signet-ring cell carcinoma of the breast, as illustrated in Figures 15.7 and 15.8, is uncommon and when the histologist is presented with a mammary

tumour of this pattern the possibility of its being a metastasis must be borne in mind[6]. In two recent reviews of carcinoma composed predominantly of signet-ring cells[7,8], both comprising 24 cases, the tumours were present in women with a mean age of 59–60 years. In the study of Hull *et al.*[7], some signet-ring cell carcinomas were associated with ductal carcinoma, some with lobular carcinoma, one with colloid carcinoma and four were pure signet-ring cell tumours. On the other hand, Merino and Livolsi[8] felt that all their cases were derived from lobular carcinoma. In each case foci of infiltrating lobular carcinoma were identified, and in 11 of the 24, lobular carcinoma *in situ* was found. Many of the cases in this study presented with advanced disease and the metastases showed a propensity to involve unusual sites, such as serosal surfaces, gastrointestinal tract, urinary tract and spleen. In both studies the mortality rate was greater as compared with other forms of mammary carcinoma. It would appear that the presence of signet-ring cells, either mixed with other variants of mammary carcinoma or in the pure form, is indicative of an unfavourable prognosis.

Secretory or Juvenile Carcinoma

As the term 'juvenile' implies, this type of mammary carcinoma was originally reported in children under the age of 15 years[9]. However, there have subsequently been several reports of secretory carcinoma in adults with a wide age range, even up to 73 years[10,11]. The tumours are usually well circumscribed and slowly growing. On histological examination the neoplasm is seen to be composed of irregular tubular structures filled with eosinophilic PAS-positive diastase-resistant material (Figures 15.9 and 15.10). In one reported case, the secretory material was identified as milk protein[12]. The malignant cells have abundant palely staining cytoplasm and, although nucleoli may be present, mitotic activity is minimal. The prognosis in children and in most adults appears to be good. So far, no deaths have been attributable to these tumours in children. However, in a recent report Tavassoli and Norris[10] reported four adult patients (21% of their series) with positive axillary nodes, one of whom died of metastatic tumour.

Lipid-rich Carcinoma

This rare type of mammary carcinoma is characterized by malignant cells with foamy cytoplasm containing a large amount of neutral lipid but no mucin (Figures 15.11 and 15.12). Lipid-rich carcinomas have been described in association both with *in situ* duct and *in situ*

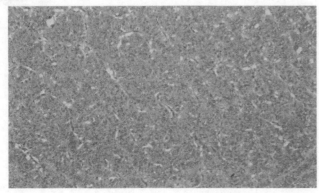

Figures 15.1 Primary carcinoid tumour of the breast. A tumour from the breast of a 45-year-old woman. Full investigation failed to reveal any evidence of a primary tumour elsewhere. The neoplasm is composed of large masses of cells which are quite regular in shape and staining properties. The stroma is scanty, but highly vascular. H & E × 96

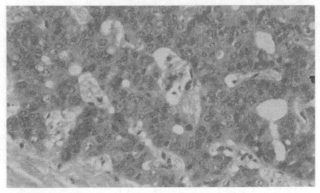

Figure 15.2 Carcinoid tumour of the breast. A neoplasm from the breast of a 43-year-old woman. The section shows masses of quite regular cells arranged as linked trabeculae. There is some fresh stromal haemorrhage, probably operative. Silver stains demonstrated argyrophil granules in many cells. H & E × 96

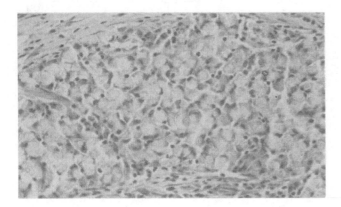

Figure 15.3 Carcinoid tumour of the breast. Section of a tumour from the breast of a 39-year-old woman. The neoplasm displays a vague glandular orientation in places. Argyrophil granules were demonstrated in the cytoplasm of a considerable number of cells. H & E × 96

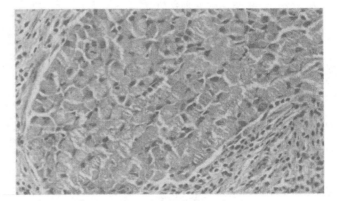

Figure 15.4 Carcinoid tumour of the breast. From the same tumour as illustrated in Figure 15.3. This high magnification shows that the neoplasm is composed of moderately sized pleomorphic cells. H & E × 240

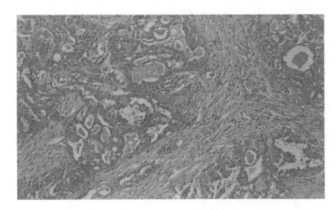

Figure 15.5 Primary carcinoid tumour of the breast. Another section of the neoplasm illustrated in Figure 15.1, stained by a silver technique and showing dark grey argyrophil granules in many of the tumour cells. Grimelius silver technique × 240

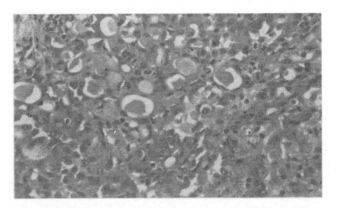

Figure 15.6 Axillary lymph node: metastasis from mammary carcinoid. From a middle-aged woman whose initial complaint was of an axillary swelling. Sometime after removal of the node, a lesion was detected in the breast. There was no evidence of a carcinoid tumour elsewhere. This section has been stained to show argyrophil granules, which are coloured brown. Grimelius silver technique counterstained with light green × 240

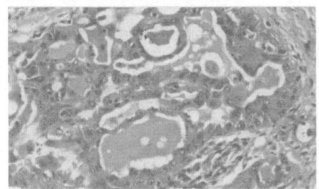

Figure 15.7 Primary signet-ring cell carcinoma of the breast. A breast tumour from a 60-year-old woman. The photomicrograph shows the neoplasm to be composed of spheroidal cells, many with palely staining, vacuolated cytoplasm, and nuclei displaced to the periphery.   H & E × 240

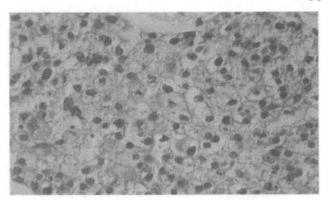

Figure 15.8 Primary signet-ring cell carcinoma of the breast. A further section of the tumour illustrated in Figure 15.6, showing abundant pink-staining intracytoplasmic mucin.   PAS after diastase digestion × 240

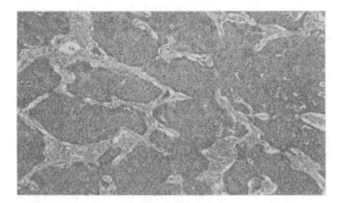

Figure 15.9 Secretory (juvenile) carcinoma. Section of a mammary tumour from a 6-year-old girl. The growth consists of irregularly shaped masses of neoplastic epithelial cells, separated by broad trabeculae of stromal fibrous tissue. Within the cell masses, there are numerous gland-like spaces filled with eosinophilic secretory material; similar material is present in the cytoplasm of some of the tumour cells.   H & E × 96

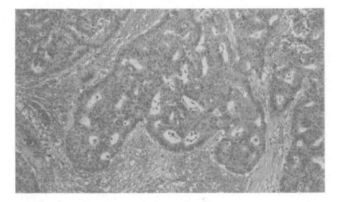

Figure 15.10 Secretory (juvenile) carcinoma. From the same tumour as that illustrated in Figure 15.9. A high magnification demonstrating the eosinophilic secretory material in the cytoplasm of some cells and in the lumina of the imperfectly formed tubular structures. The material is PAS-positive and diastase resistant.   H & E × 240

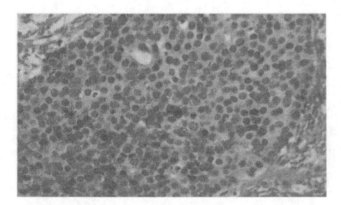

Figure 15.11 Lipid-rich carcinoma of the breast. A mammary carcinoma composed of closely packed spheroidal cells, with hyperchromatic nuclei and abundant, vacuolated, foamy cytoplasm. Frozen sections of unembedded tumour tissue, stained with Oil Red O, showed abundant lipid in almost all the cells.   H & E × 240

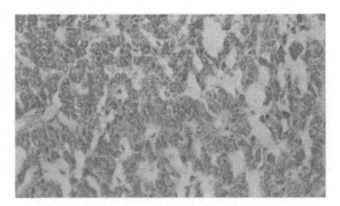

Figure 15.12 Lipid-rich carcinoma of the breast. From the same tumour as that illustrated in Figure 15.11. This shows an intraductal component and demonstrates the abundant intracytoplasmic lipid (stained red) in the carcinoma cells.   Frozen section, stained with Oil Red O × 240

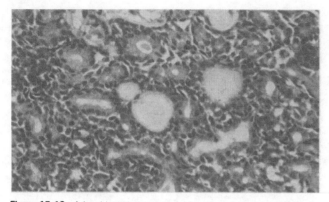

Figure 15.13 Adenoid cystic carcinoma of the breast. A tumour from the breast of a 48-year-old woman. The neoplasm is composed of darkly-staining spheroidal and polyhedral cells with relatively scanty cytoplasm. Both the cribriform (pseudocystic) spaces and true glandular lumina are evident. The cribriform spaces display circumferential rings of hyaline eosinophilic material. Electron microscopic studies indicate that the spaces contain basement membrane material.   H & E × 96

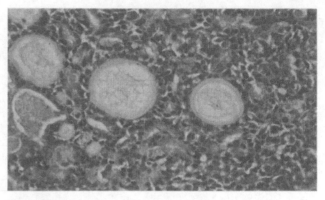

Figure 15.14 Adenoid cystic carcinoma of the breast. Another part of the tumour illustrated in Figure 15.13. Both the cribriform pattern and cribriform spaces are again seen. Special stains show mucoid material in the large spaces to be PAS-negative while PAS-positive material is present in the smaller glandular lumina.   H & E × 96

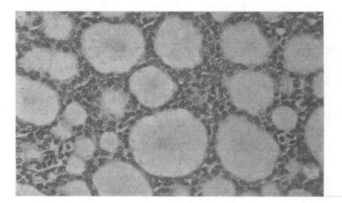

Figure 15.15 Adenoid cystic carcinoma of the breast. A tumour from the breast of a 59-year-old woman. The neoplasm is composed of regular spheroidal cells, with a characteristic cribriform pattern. The spaces contain mucinous material, staining palely with haematoxylin.   H & E × 240

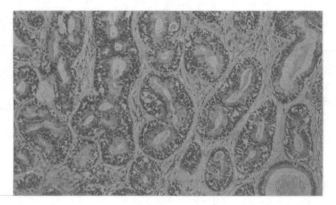

Figure 15.16 Adenoid cystic carcinoma of the breast. In this field there is prominent tubule formation with both columnar juxtaluminal cells and thick myoepithelial mantles. In other parts the tumour displayed a typical cribriform pattern (Figures 15.13 and 15.14).   H & E × 96

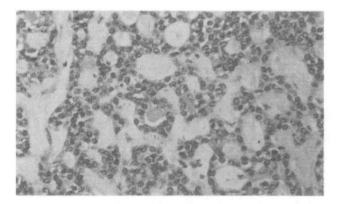

Figure 15.17 Adenoid cystic carcinoma of the breast. Another part of the neoplasm shown in Figure 15.15. In this area some of the cribriform spaces intercommunicate. Just below and to the left of centre, there is a glandular lumen containing eosinophilic secretion, such material is strongly PAS-positive.   H & E × 240

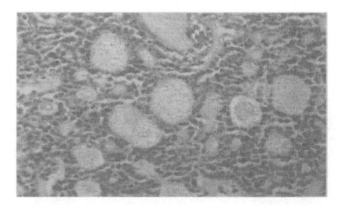

Figure 15.18 Adenoid cystic carcinoma of the breast. A further section of the tumour illustrated in Figures 15.15 and 15.17. The material in the cribriform spaces stains intensely with Alcian blue.   Alcian blue/neutral red × 240

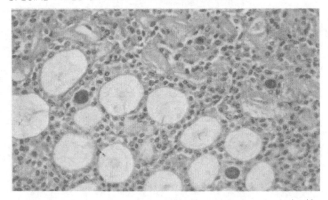

Figure 15.19 Adenoid cystic carcinoma of the breast. A section stained by the periodic acid-Schiff technique after diastase digestion. The material within the cribriform spaces stains very palely, but there are a number of small glandular lumina containing strongly PAS-positive mucin.   PAS after diastase digestion × 240

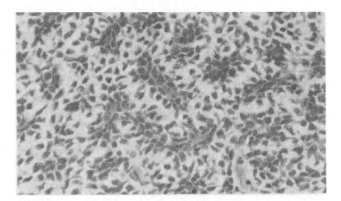

Figure 15.20 Adenoid cystic carcinoma of the breast. This section shows another microscopic pattern, in which small tubular structures, containing PAS-positive secretions, are surrounded by loosely-arranged, rounded or angulated cells which are probably myoepithelial.   PAS after diastase digestion × 240

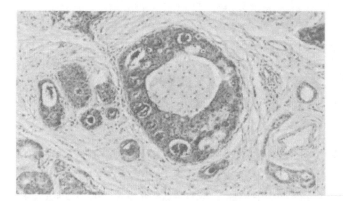

Figure 15.21 Cribriform intraduct carcinoma. A section stained by the PAS technique, illustrating the strongly positive reaction of the mucin in the cribriform spaces. Compare this with the adenoid cystic carcinoma shown in Figure 15.19.   PAS after diastase digestion × 96

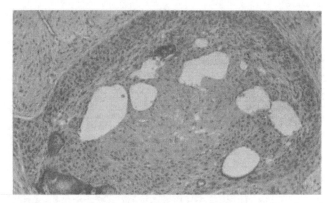

Figure 15.22 Mammary carcinoma with mucoepidermoid pattern. Part of an infiltrating carcinoma, composed of large masses of cohesive tumour cells, displaying squamous traits and also pools of basophilic mucin. The mucin stained red in both PAS and mucicarmine preparations.   H & E × 96

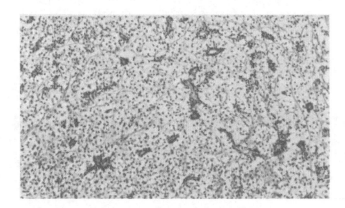

Figure 15.23 Mammary tumour with the structure of a clear-cell hidradenoma. Sections of a sharply circumscribed tumour excised from the breast of 24-year-old woman. The growth was situated deeply and was not attached to skin. Two cell types are apparent: darkly-staining juxtaluminal cells forming tubules, and surrounding cells with abundant clear cytoplasm. The clear cells are probably myoepithelial; their cytoplasm contains abundant glycogen.   H & E × 96

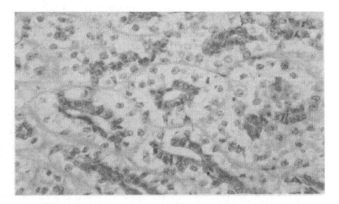

Figure 15.24 Mammary tumour with the structure of a clear-cell hidradenoma. Higher magnification of the section illustrated in Figure 15.23. There is a striking contrast between the darkly-stained juxtaluminal cells and the clear cells which form mantles around them.   H & E × 240

lobular carcinoma[13]. Van Bogaert and Maldague[14] divided lipid-secreting carcinoma into three groups: a histiocytoid type, a sebaceous type and carcinoma with apocrine extrusion of nuclei.

Fisher et al.[15], in a study of the lipid content of a series of consecutive breast cancers, found lipid to be present in a very high proportion and in almost one third it was assessed as being moderate or marked in amount. They did not find that the presence of lipid correlated with the typical description of so-called lipid-rich mammary carcinoma. They did find, however, that the presence of a moderate or marked amount of lipid was associated with significantly more squamous metaplasia, anaplasia and high histological grades. There was also a suggestion that the amount of lipid correlated with short term treatment failure. This is in keeping with the study of Ramos and Taylor[13], who reported a 50% mortality in the 2 years following diagnosis of lipid-rich carcinoma.

Some carcinomas with abundant clear cytoplasm contain large amounts of glycogen rather than lipid. Such glycogen-rich tumours have been described as a separate entity[16].

Histiocytoid Carcinoma

This term has been used by Hood and colleagues[17] to describe a variant of metastatic carcinoma of the breast composed of clumps of cells with small nuclei and abundant pale cytoplasm which resemble histiocytes on cursory examination. In the cases reported by Hood et al. the metastatic lesions were all in the eyelids. Of their 13 cases of carcinoma of the breast metastatic to the eyelid, eight were of histiocytoid pattern and seven presented diagnostic problems histologically. The diagnostic difficulty was compounded by the fact that in five of the eight the metastasis was the presenting symptom of the disease. The cells of histiocytoid carcinoma contain mucin and its demonstration may be of diagnostic value. The tumours are probably a variant of lobular carcinoma.

Adenoid Cystic Carcinoma

Adenoid cystic carcinoma is a rare type of mammary tumour. Although histologically identical to adenoid cystic carcinoma of the salivary glands, it is associated with a much more favourable prognosis. In a review of the literature on nearly 100 cases, Anthony and James[18] found no characteristic age distribution for patients with adenoid cystic carcinoma of the breast. The tumour is usually seen in women, although examples in men have been described. The duration of symptoms is frequently long, the tumour usually presenting as a mass in the breast and often arising in the nipple area; pain and tenderness appear to be frequent symptoms. Most of the tumours are between 1 and 3 cm in maximal diameter, but occasionally they are larger. On gross examination, adenoid cystic carcinoma is usually fairly well defined, sometimes lobulated and occasionally cystic. Microscopically, multiple cyst-like spaces are surrounded by relatively uniform basaloid cells, probably myoepithelial in type, producing a cribriform pattern (Figures 15.13–15.17). Ultrastructural studies show that these spaces are extracellular compartments lined by a basement membrane[19]; they contain acid mucopolysaccaride which is Alcian blue positive, but stains only faintly with PAS (Figures 15.18 and 15.19). In addition to these

cribriform spaces, there are scattered smaller duct-like structures which contain PAS-positive material (Figures 15.19 and 15.20). Thus there is a mixture of pseudocystic spaces lined by basaloid cells and true glandular lumina lined by epithelial cells. Mitoses are rare and necrosis absent. Perineural invasion is often present and some authors believe that this accounts for the tenderness frequently described. It is important to distinguish this type of tumour from the much more common cribriform intraductal carcinoma with which it is sometimes confused[18,20]. In the latter the cystic spaces all contain strongly PAS-positive material (Figure 15.21).

There have been occasional reports of lymph node metastases from adenoid cystic carcinoma and of patients dying with disseminated disease, but some of these cases are not well documented. Local recurrence has been recorded in a few cases but does not apparently alter the favourable prognosis[18,19].

Other Tumours Microscopically Similar to Those of Salivary or Sweat Gland Origin

The most common example of a mammary tumour similar to those of salivary or sweat gland origin is adenoid cystic carcinoma; however, a few other such tumours occasionally occur and merit brief mention here.

Pleomorphic Adenoma (Mixed Tumour)

Pleomorphic adenoma is the term currently preferred for the common salivary gland tumour. When arising in the skin it is often designated mixed tumour or chondroid syringoma. In a recent study, Makek and von Hochstetter[21] reported three cases of pleomorphic adenoma of the human breast and reviewed a further 15 examples from the literature. The age at operation ranged from 23 to 78 years; the one male patient included was 60 years old. Most of the tumours measured between 1 and 4 cm in diameter, but one of 20 cm has been recorded. Malignant change has not been observed although these mammary tumours, like their salivary gland counterparts, may recur locally. Microscopically, pleomorphic adenoma displays tubules with myoepithelial mantles, hyaline stroma, and myxoid, chondroid and osseous areas. Electron microscopic studies confirm that the stromal cells are myoepithelial in type[22]. Foci of calcification may occur within the ducts. The neoplasms have to be distinguished from carcinoma of the breast with stromal metaplasia and from mammary sarcoma. Although pleomorphic adenoma of the breast is rare, the importance of its recognition is emphasized by the fact that unnecessarily aggressive operations have occasionally been performed on patients with these tumours.

Mucoepidermoid Tumour

Two cases of low grade mucoepidermoid carcinoma of the breast were reported by Patchefsky and colleagues[23]. The patients were women of 66 and 70 years of age. Microscopically the neoplasms were morphologically identical to low grade mucoepidermoid carcinoma of the salivary glands and displayed sheets of polygonal cells merging with squamous and sharply defined mucinous elements (Figure 15.22); there was evidence of origin within the mammary ducts. It was suggested that these growths were indolent breast tumours analogous in their behaviour to those of the salivary glands. A case of high grade mucoepidermoid carcinoma of the breast in a 46-year-old woman has been described by Kovi et al.[24]. The patient was treated by radical mastectomy and 17 of 19 axillary nodes contained metastatic tumour.

Clear Cell Hidradenoma and Eccrine Spiradenoma

Six cases of clear cell hidradenoma originating in the breast were reported by Finck et al.[25]. Five of the patients were women aged between 30 and 60 years and one was a 42-year-old man. The largest tumour measured 4 cm across. Four arose superficially beneath the nipple and areola; two were situated deep in the breast. The authors suggested that clear cell hidradenoma of the breast is closely related to papilloma of the mammary ducts. Microscopically, the tumours are morphologically identical to those arising in the skin (Figures 15.23 and 15.24).

Draheim and colleagues[26] reported an unusual tumour of the breast resembling an eccrine spiradenoma. The patient was a 44-year-old woman and the tumour measured 2.5 cm along its greatest dimension. There was a recurrence 16 months after local removal.

References

1. Cubilla, A. I. and Woodruff, J. M. (1977). Primary carcinoid tumour of the breast. A report of eight patients. Am. J. Surg. Pathol., 1, 283

2. Kaneko, H., Hojo, H., Ishikawa, S., Yamanouchi, H., Sumida, T. and Saito, R. (1978). Norepinephrine-producing tumours of bilateral breasts. A case report. Cancer, 41, 2002

3. Taxy, J. B., Tischler, A. S., Insalaco, S. J. and Battifora, H. (1981). 'Carcinoid' tumour of the breast. A variant of conventional breast cancer? Hum. Pathol., 12, 170

4. Azzopardi, J. G., Muretto, P., Goddeeris, P., Eusebi, V. and Lauweryns, J. M. (1982). 'Carcinoid' tumours of the breast: the morphological spectrum of argyrophil carcinomas. Histopathology, 6, 549

5. Clayton, F., Sibley, R. K., Ordonez, N. G. and Hanssen, G. (1982). Argyrophilic breast carcinomas. Evidence of lactational differentiation. Am. J. Surg. Pathol., 6, 323

6. Harris, M., Wells, S. and Vasudev, K. S. (1978). Primary signet ring cell carcinoma of the breast. Histopathology, 2, 171

7. Hull, M. T., Seo, I. S., Battersby, J. S. and Csicsko, J. F. (1980). Signet-ring cell carcinoma of the breast. A clinicopathologic study of 24 cases. Am. J. Clin. Pathol., 73, 31

8. Merino, M. J. and Livolsi, V. A. (1981). Signet ring carcinoma of the female breast: a clinicopathologic analysis of 24 cases. Cancer, 48, 1830

9. McDivitt, R. W. and Stewart, F. W. (1966). Breast carcinoma in children. J. Am. Med. Assoc. 195, 388

10. Tavassoli, F. A. and Norris, H. J. (1980). Secretory carcinoma of the breast. Cancer, 45, 2404

11. Oberman, H. A. (1980). Secretory carcinoma of the breast in adults. Am. J. Surg. Pathol., 4, 465

12. Botta, G., Fessia, L. and Ghiringhello, B. (1982). Juvenile milk protein secreting carcinoma. Virchows Arch. [Pathol. Anat.], 395, 145

13. Ramos, C. V. and Taylor, H. B. (1974). Lipid-rich carcinoma of the breast. A clinicopathologic analysis of 13 examples. Cancer, 33, 812

14. van Bogaert, L.-J. and Maldague, P. (1977). Histologic variants of lipid-secreting carcinoma of breast. Virchows Arch. A. Pathol. Anat. Histol., 375, 345

15. Fisher, E. R., Gregorio, R., Kim, W. S. and Redmond, C. (1977). Lipid in invasive cancer of the breast. Am. J. Clin. Pathol., 68, 558

16. Hull, M. T., Priest, J. B., Broadie, T. A., Ransburg, R. C. and McCarthy, L. J. (1981). Glycogen-rich clear cell carcinoma of the breast: a light and electron microscopic study. Cancer, 48, 2003

17. Hood, C. I., Font, R. L. and Zimmerman, L. E. (1973). Metastatic mammary carcinoma in the eyelid with histiocytoid appearance. Cancer, 31, 793

18. Anthony, P. P. and James, P. D. (1975). Adenoid cystic carcinoma of the breast: prevalence, diagnostic criteria, and histogenesis. J. Clin. Pathol., 28, 647

19. Qizilbash, A. H., Patterson, M. C. and Oliveira, K. F. (1977). Adenoid cystic carcinoma of the breast. Arch. Pathol. Lab. Med., 101, 302

20. Harris, M. (1977). Pseudoadenoid cystic carcinoma of the breast. Arch. Pathol. Lab. Med., 101, 307

21. Makek, M. and von Hochstetter, A. R. (1980). Pleomorphic adenoma of the human breast. J. Surg. Oncol., 14, 281

22. McClure, J., Smith, P. S. and Jamieson, G. G. (1982). 'Mixed' salivary type adenoma of the human female breast. Arch. Pathol. Lab. Med., 106, 615

23. Patchefsky, A. S., Frauenhoffer, C. M., Krall, R. A. and Cooper, H. S. (1979). Low-grade mucoepidermoid carcinoma of the breast. Arch. Pathol. Lab. Med., 103, 196

24. Kovi, J., Duong, H. D. and Leffall, L. D. Jr. (1981). High-grade mucoepidermoid carcinoma of the breast. Arch. Pathol. Lab. Med., 105, 612

25. Finck, F. M., Schwinn, C. P. and Keasbey, L. E. (1968). Clear cell hidradenoma of the breast. Cancer, 22, 125

26. Draheim, J. H., Neubecker, R. D. and Sprinz, H. (1959). An unusual tumour of the breast resembling eccrine spiradenoma. Am. J. Clin. Pathol., 31, 511

Squamous Cell Carcinoma

Pure squamous cell carcinoma of the breast is rare. Focal squamous metaplasia, however, is not uncommon in infiltrating duct carcinoma and is seen relatively frequently in medullary carcinoma with lymphoid stroma. There are also a few reports of squamous carcinoma arising in a cystosarcoma phyllodes tumour[1,2]. Tumours of the skin and nipple appendages should not be confused with mammary squamous cell carcinoma. Toikkanen[3] in a recent review found only three pure squamous cell carcinomas amongst 4000 cases of primary carcinoma of the breast. The tumours are usually large with a central cystic cavity lined by obvious squamous epithelium (Figure 16.1). Areas of marked pleomorphism are common and spindle cell areas are often present. However, some authorities[1] distinguish between squamous cell carcinoma with spindle cell dedifferentiation and pure squamous cell carcinoma without spindle cell change which they consider to be another form of metaplasia. Sometimes dissociation of the cells in a squamous cell carcinoma gives rise to a pattern resembling an angiosarcoma (Figure 16.2). The demonstration of reticulin is of value in distinguishing a tumour with such a pattern from a true sarcoma, because in squamous cell carcinoma the reticulin fibres are usually present only in relation to stromal blood vessels (Figure 16.3).

There is some controversy regarding the prognosis of mammary squamous cell carcinoma and its age incidence. The tumour has usually been considered to have a poor prognosis and to occur in women older than those with other forms of mammary carcinoma. Azzopardi[1], however, maintains that discrepancies in the literature regarding the prognosis and age of the patients with this type of tumour are due to failure to differentiate between pure squamous cell carcinoma, other types of mammary carcinoma with squamous metaplasia, squamous cell carcinomas arising in a pre-existing tumour and squamous cell carcinoma with spindle cell metaplasia.

Sarcomatoid Carcinoma (Pseudosarcoma)

Dedifferentiation of an infiltrating duct carcinoma may result in a spindle cell tumour with a sarcomatoid pattern, and lead to an erroneous diagnosis of sarcoma (Figures 16.4 and 16.5). However, careful examination of multiple sections will usually reveal transitions from an obvious epithelial tumour, sometimes of squamous type, to the pseudosarcomatous growth[1,4].

Carcinoma with Bone and Cartilage Formation

Bone and cartilage formation in mammary carcinoma is uncommon. Although metaplastic carcinoma of the breast is usually considered to occur in elderly patients, this is not borne out by the study of Huvos et al.[5], in which the mean age was similar to that of patients with conventional forms of mammary carcinoma. On average these tumours tend to be large and to behave in an aggressive fashion. This was emphasized by Huvos and co-workers[5], who found that patients with tumours showing bone and cartilage formation had a poorer prognosis than those demonstrating squamous and spindle cell metaplasia. Metaplastic changes resulting in bone and cartilage formation, as shown in Figures 16.6–16.9, have been reported in association with infiltrating duct carcinoma, medullary carcinoma with lymphoid stroma and infiltrating lobular carcinoma[5]. Transition from the carcinoma to the heterologous element can usually be demonstrated[6]. Metastases occur more commonly via the bloodstream than by lymphatics, and the metastatic deposits consist of pure carcinoma without the heterologous elements[5].

Apocrine Carcinoma

Mammary carcinomas containing malignant cells with abundant eosinophilic cytoplasm having a superficial resemblance to apocrine cells are not uncommon (Figure 16.10). However, true apocrine differentiation is rare, even in focal parts of a tumour, and is only seen in about 1% of all mammary carcinomas[7]. Pure apocrine carcinoma is extremely unusual[1]. There is no evidence that the presence of apocrine change has any prognostic significance.

Carcinoma with Osteoclast-like (Epulis-like) Giant Cells in the Stroma

Multinucleated osteoclast-like giant cells have been described within the stroma of infiltrating duct and lobular carcinomas[8-10]. Haemorrhage and marked vascularity are often noted within the stroma of these tumours. Giant cells similar to those present within the primary tumour have also been seen in lymph node and visceral metastases[10]. These giant cells are benign and should be distinguished from tumour giant cells, including those of malignant giant cell tumour of soft parts, which has been rarely reported in the breast[9]. Osteoclast-like giant cells can also occur in metaplastic tumours containing bone and cartilage. The limited follow-up information on carcinomas with osteoclast-like giant cells in the stroma precludes prognostic evaluation.

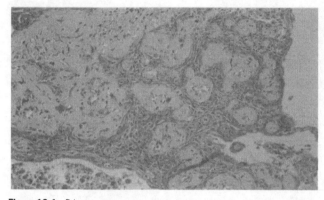

Figure 16.1 Primary squamous cell carcinoma of the breast. An example of a 'pure' squamous cell mammary carcinoma. The tumour formed a mass several centimetres in diameter. Bisection revealed a central cystic cavity surrounded by pinkish-grey, solid neoplastic tissue. This photomicrograph shows part of the cyst wall which is lined by well-differentiated, neoplastic, stratified squamous epithelium. H & E × 96

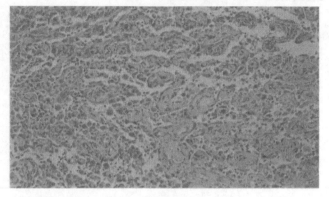

Figure 16.2 Primary squamous cell carcinoma of the breast. Another part of the tumour illustrated in Figure 16.1. Here the growth is poorly differentiated and there is marked dissociation of the carcinoma cells, both from each other and from the supporting stroma. H & E × 96

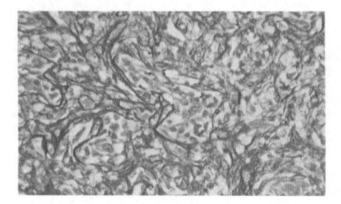

Figure 16.3 Primary squamous cell carcinoma of the breast. Sections of a very cellular and poorly differentiated part of a squamous cell carcinoma, demonstrating reticulin fibres surrounding groups of tumour cells rather than forming a pericellular network – an epithelial rather than a mesenchymal pattern. Silver impregnation for reticulin/neutral red × 240

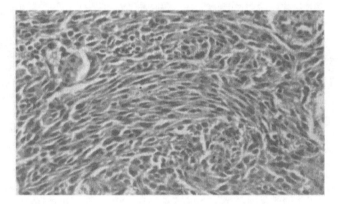

Figure 16.4 Carcinoma of the breast with undifferentiated spindle cell component. Section of a mammary tumour from a 64-year-old woman. The photomicrograph shows closely packed, spindle shaped neoplastic cells, cut both longitudinally and transversely. In other parts, the tumour had the more conventional pattern of an infiltrating duct carcinoma. The spindle shaped cells are considered to be carcinomatous, not sarcomatous. H & E × 240

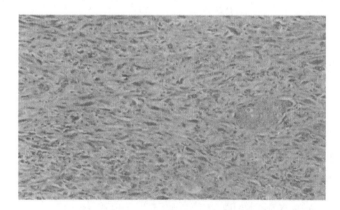

Figure 16.5 Carcinoma of the breast with undifferentiated spindle cell (sarcomatoid) component. A small island of cohesive cells, clearly epithelial in type, can be seen towards the right edge of the field. The rest of the tumour in the photomicrograph consists of spindle shaped cells with pleomorphic nuclei and eosinophilic cytoplasm: an appearance which may give a false impression of a myogenic neoplasm. H & E × 96

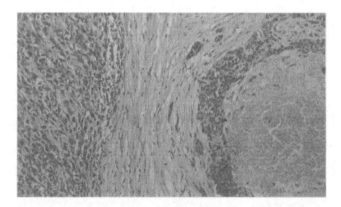

Figure 16.6 Carcinoma of the breast, with an osteosarcomatous component. Section of a mammary tumour from a 56-year-old woman. On the right, there is part of the carcinoma showing comedo-type necrosis. On the left, there is a very cellular neoplastic component, displaying many mitotic figures; this tissue merged with the osteoblastic growth illustrated in Figures 16.7 and 16.8. H & E × 96

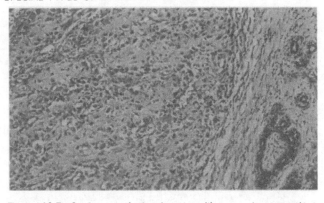

Figure 16.7 Carcinoma of the breast, with an osteosarcomatous component. Another part of the tumour illustrated in Figure 16.6, showing the sarcomatous component with osteoid formation. A few mammary ductules are seen on the extreme right.   H & E × 96

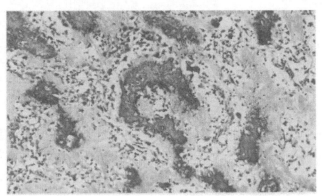

Figure 16.8 Carcinoma of the breast, with an osteosarcomatous component. From the same tumour as that illustrated in Figures 16.6 and 16.7. This section shows the sarcomatous component, featuring abundant neoplastic osteoid and bone.   H & E × 96

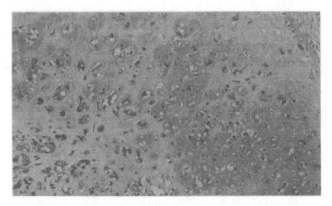

Figure 16.9 Carcinoma of the breast with chondroid component. A tumour showing pleomorphic hyperchromatic tumour cells, particularly in the left half of the field, and a well developed chondroid pattern in the right half. H & E × 96

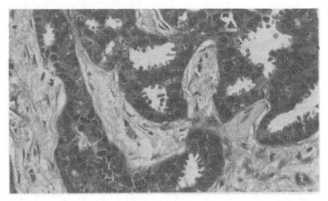

Figure 16.10 Infiltrating carcinoma with apocrine traits. Sections of an infiltrating mammary carcinoma, featuring cells with pleomorphic nuclei and brightly eosinophilic cytoplasm. The tumour cells also display glandular orientation with cytoplasmic protrusions ('apocrine snouts') into the lumina of the tubules.   H & E × 240

Infiltrating Papillary Carcinoma

Although a papillary pattern is not uncommon in intraductal carcinomas, infiltrating tumours with predominantly papillary pattern are rare. Fisher and colleagues[11] found only 35 examples amongst 1603 cases of invasive mammary carcinoma. Papillary carcinoma is a variant of infiltrating duct carcinoma and is usually associated with a relatively good prognosis (see Chapter 12).

Carcinoma in Children

Mammary carcinoma in childhood is a rare occurrence. The characteristic type seen most frequently in this age group is the secretory carcinoma already described. Very occasionally, other conventional types of mammary carcinoma occur in children and these may have a less favourable prognosis[1,12].

Carcinoma of the Male Breast

Carcinoma of the male breast is rare, accounting for about 1% of all breast carcinomas in both sexes. Men tend to develop the disease at a slightly older age than women and the history is usually longer[13-15]. Male breast cancer has traditionally been associated with a poor prognosis, which according to some authorities is related to the fact that men often present with more advanced tumours than women. Tumours of the male breast are generally centrally located, and rapidly involve skin and underlying structures, and permeation of the subareolar lymphatics leads to early involvement of regional nodes[14]. However, other authorities claim that there is no difference in the incidence of different stages of the disease between men and women at the time of presentation and that the prognosis is comparable to that of cancer of the female breast[13,15]. Heller et al.[14] found that the poorer prognosis in men was limited to those with pathologically positive lymph nodes. They felt that the low survival rate of men with breast cancer was due to some other factor that increased the lethality of the cancer metastatic to axillary nodes, and not to a predominance of advanced disease.

Microscopically, invasive carcinoma of the male breast is similar to that in women. All types of carcinoma have been reported in the male, including very rare cases of lobular carcinoma[16]. The rarity of lobular carcinoma is to be expected, since lobules are not normally present in the male breast. As in women, the most common type is infiltrating duct carcinoma. Paget's disease of the male nipple has also been reported[14].

There is a dispute concerning the relationship of gynaecomastia to breast cancer. Although it may be diagnosed microscopically in a relatively high proportion of patients[16], it is generally held that mammary carcinoma usually develops in the absence of clinical gynaecomastia. However, an increased incidence of carcinoma has been reported in men with Klinefelter's syndrome[1].

References

1. Azzopardi, J.G. (1979). *Problems in Breast Pathology*, p. 258. (Vol. 11 in Bennington, J.L. (consulting ed.) *Major Problems in Pathology*.) (London, Philadelphia and Toronto: Saunders)

2. Cornog, J.L., Mobini, J., Steiger, E. and Enterline, H.T., (1971). Squamous carcinoma of the breast. *Am. J. Clin. Pathol.*, **55**, 410–417

3. Toikkanen, S. (1981). Primary squamous cell carcinoma of the breast. *Cancer*, **48**, 1629–1632

4. Gersell, D.J. and Katzenstein, A.-L.A. (1981). Spindle cell carcinoma of the breast. *Hum. Pathol.*, **12**, 550–561

5. Huvos, A.G., Lucas, J.C. Jr. and Foote, F.W. (1973). Metaplastic breast carcinoma. NY *State J. Med.*, **73**, 1078–1082

6. Kahn, L.B., Uys, C.J., Dale, J. and Rutherfoord, S. (1978). Carcinoma of the breast with metaplasia to chondrosarcoma: a light and electron microscopic study. *Histopathology*, **2**, 93–106

7. Frable, W.J. and Kay, S. (1968). Carcinoma of the breast. Histologic and clinical features of apocrine tumours. *Cancer*, **21**, 756–763

8. Agnantis, N.T. and Rosen, P.P. (1979). Mammary carcinoma with osteoclast-like giant cells. *Am. J. Clin. Pathol.*, **72**, 383–389

9. Factor, S.M., Biempica, L., Ratner, I., Ahuja, K.K. and Biempica, S. (1977). Carcinoma of the breast with multinucleated reactive stromal giant cells. *Virchows Arch. A. Pathol. Anat. Histol.*, **374**, 1–12

10. Levin, A., Rywlin, A.M. and Tachmes, P. (1981). Carcinoma of the breast with stromal epulis-like giant cells. *South. Med. J.*, **74**, 889–891

11. Fisher, E.R., Palekar, A.S., Redmond, C., Barton, B. and Fisher B. (1980). Pathologic findings from the National Surgical Adjuvant Breast Project (Protocol No. 4). VI. Invasive papillary cancer. *Am. J. Clin. Pathol.*, **73**, 313–321.

12. Ashikari, H., Jun, M.Y., Farrow, J.H., Rosen, P.P. and Johnston, S.F. (1977). Breast carcinoma in children and adolescents. *Clin. Bull.*, **7**, 55–62

13. Yap, H.Y., Tashima, C.K., Blumenschein, G.R. and Eckles, N.E. (1979). Male breast cancer. *Cancer*, **44**, 748–754

14. Heller, K.S., Rosen, P.P., Schottenfeld, D., Ashikari, R. and Kinne, D.W. (1978). Male breast cancer. A clinicopathological study of 97 cases. *Ann. Surg.*, **188**, 60–64

15. Carlsson, G., Hafstrom, L. and Jonsson, P.-E. (1981). Male breast cancer. *Clin. Oncol.*, **7**, 149–155

16. Giffler, R.F. and Kay, S. (1976). Small-cell carcinoma of the male mammary gland. *Am. J. Clin. Pathol.*, **66**, 715–722

Paget's Disease of the Nipple

Paget's disease of the nipple presents as a red, weeping, often partly crusting eczematoid lesion (Figure 17.1), and clinical differentiation from eczema is often impossible. It is present in about 1–2% of patients with mammary carcinoma and is occasionally seen in the male breast. In 99% of patients with Paget's disease a carcinoma can be demonstrated pathologically in the underlying breast, although in over half of the patients the tumour is clinically impalpable. The tumour associated with Paget's disease may be either a pure *in situ* duct carcinoma or an infiltrating duct tumour. The association of Paget's disease with pure lobular carcinoma is rare. The prognosis for patients with Paget's disease but no palpable neoplasm is considerably more favourable than for those in whom the tumour is clinically overt[1-3]. This is probably because many of the impalpable carcinomas are *in situ*[1,2]. The underlying carcinoma is sometimes very small and may only involve a single lactiferous duct (Figures 17.2 and 17.3).

The histogenesis of Paget's disease remains controversial. There is disagreement as to whether Paget cells originate from an underlying mammary carcinoma and spread upwards through the ductal epithelium to the nipple, or whether they arise within the epidermis as part of a widespread *in situ* malignant change affecting at one and the same time both the ductal epithelium and the epidermis.

The typical microscopic appearance of mammary Paget's disease is shown in Figures 17.4–17.8. The epidermis of the nipple is permeated by neoplastic cells with large nuclei, prominent nucleoli and abundant palely-staining cytoplasm, which frequently contains PAS-positive droplets (Figure 17.6). These cells (sometimes called Paget cells) are disposed singly or in small groups and occasionally show an acinar arrangement. They tend to shrink with fixation and often appear to lie within vacuoles (Figure 17.7). The Paget cells may be few in number lying mainly in the malpighian layer, or so abundant that they extensively replace and destroy the epidermis (Figure 17.8). The sub-adjacent dermis displays telangiectasia and inflammatory cell infiltration. Direct invasion of the epidermis by malignant cells from an underlying infiltrating carcinoma, as shown in Figure 17.9, should not be confused with Paget's disease. Another condition sometimes mistaken for Paget's disease is illustrated in Figure 17.10. The *'cellules claires'* illustrated here are occasionally seen within the nipple epithelium. Although uncommon in the nipple, Bowen's disease and malignant melanoma of the superficial spreading ('pagetoid') type should also be considered in the differential diagnosis. The presence of PAS-positive intracytoplasmic mucin is helpful in confirming the diagnosis of Paget's disease, but unfortunately not all Paget cells are PAS-positive. In Bowen's disease, although some cells may contain PAS-positive material within their cytoplasm, most of this, apart from a few small granules is diastase labile. Moreover this material does not react positively with other mucin stains. Multinucleated cells and individual-cell keratinization are often seen in Bowen's disease, and, when present, are of diagnostic value. Distinction from the 'pagetoid' type of malignant melanoma may be more difficult, particularly as Paget cells occasionally contain melanin pigment (Figure 17.11). In melanoma, some of the tumour cells border directly onto and invade the dermis, whereas Paget cells generally remain entirely within the epidermis, even when the disease is advanced.

The pathological appearance of Paget's disease is sometimes seen in the absence of the clinical manifestation when sections of the nipple are taken from mastectomy specimens. As might be expected, such patients do not have the favourable outlook seen in patients with clinical Paget's disease and an impalpable tumour and, indeed, appear to do worse than the average patient with breast cancer[4].

Inflammatory Carcinoma of the Breast

Like Paget's disease of the nipple, inflammatory carcinoma is not a particular histopathological type of carcinoma but rather a pattern of spread which produces a characteristic clinical appearance. Inflammatory carcinoma of the breast is not common, occurring in less than 2% of patients with breast cancer[5-7]. It is seen in no particular age group. The involved breast is warm, usually red and oedematous and, although a localized mass may be palpable, quite frequently the breast is diffusely involved by tumour. In the vast majority of clinical cases of inflammatory carcinoma, evidence of extensive dermal lymphatic permeation is seen on pathological examination (Figure 17.12) and it is this, rather than the inflammatory appearance *per se*, which is the significant feature indicating incurability by surgery. The term 'dermal lymphatic carcinomatosis' has been suggested as an alternative to 'inflammatory carcinoma' to emphasize this point[5]. The prognosis is poor, with few patients surviving more than 5 years.

Although the pathological appearance of widespread dermal lymphatic infiltration may occur in the absence of the clinical picture of inflammatory carcinoma, this is rare, and it appears that the patients have the same poor prognosis as those with the typical clinical manifestations. However, there is some controversy concerning the treatment and prognosis of the very small proportion of patients who present with the clinical picture of inflammatory carcinoma but without pathologically identifiable dermal lymphatic permeation[6,7].

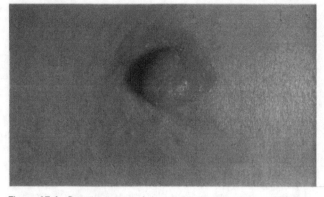

Figure 17.1 Paget's disease of the nipple. Clinical photograph showing erythema of the nipple and areola, with some surface exudation and crusting

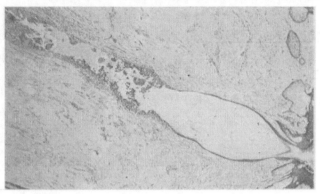

Figure 17.2 *In situ* carcinoma of lactiferous duct, associated with Paget's disease. The patient had the typical clinical and histological features of Paget's disease of the nipple. Examination of the mastectomy specimen revealed *in situ* carcinoma affecting the large lactiferous duct shown here. The carcinoma involves the duct in the left half of the field; to the right the duct becomes somewhat dilated before reaching the skin surface at the extreme right-hand bottom corner of the photograph.   H & E × 24

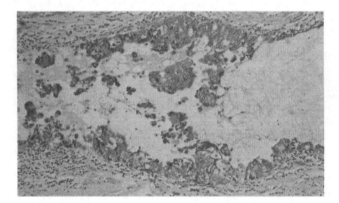

Figure 17.3 Intraduct carcinoma associated with Paget's disease. Higher magnification of the *in situ* carcinoma involving the lactiferous duct illustrated in Figure 17.2.   H & E × 96

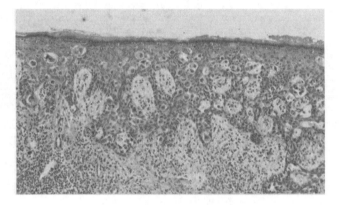

Figure 17.4 Paget's disease of the nipple. Section of nipple skin showing numerous large neoplastic (Paget) cells scattered through the epidermis. There is a lymphocytic infiltrate in the superficial dermis. The keratinocytes are maturing normally to form the stratum corneum.   H & E × 96

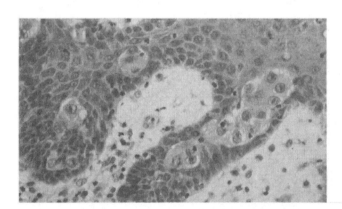

Figure 17.5 Paget's disease of the nipple. The large Paget cells have palely-staining cytoplasm and moderately prominent nucleoli. They are arranged as clusters which are sharply demarcated from the surrounding keratinocytes.   H & E × 240

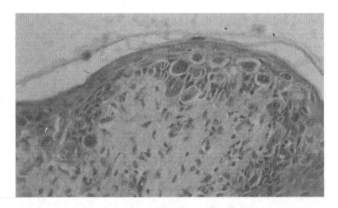

Figure 17.6 Paget's disease of the nipple. Sections showing intracytoplasmic mucin (stained red) in the cytoplasm of the Paget cells. Only some of the cells contain mucin, so a positive staining reaction may not be obtained in small biopsy specimens.   PAS after diastase digestion × 96

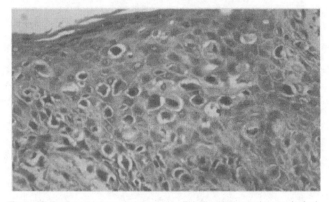

Figure 17.7 Paget's disease of the nipple. This illustrates another cytological pattern in Paget's disease. The neoplastic cells appear to have shrunk away from the adjacent keratinocytes, and their nuclei are hyperchromatic and distorted: probably a degenerative phenomenon. H & E × 240

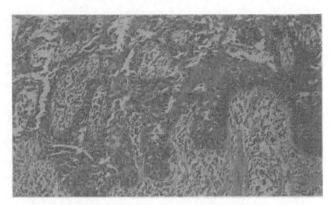

Figure 17.8 Paget's disease of the nipple. This illustrates a more advanced stage of the disease when the epidermis has become extensively disorganized by the infiltrating Paget cells. The dermis is oedematous and is infiltrated with lymphocytes and plasmacytes. H & E × 96

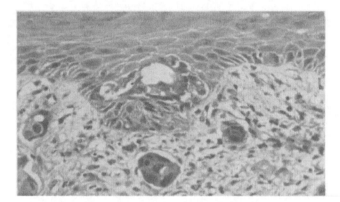

Figure 17.9 Invasion of dermis and epidermis by breast cancer. Small clusters of carcinoma cells are present in the dermis and epidermis. This represents direct invasion of the skin from an underlying cancer of the breast. The lesion is morphologically and pathogenetically distinct from Paget's disease. H & E × 240

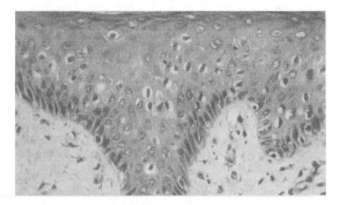

Figure 17.10 Nipple skin; 'clear-cell' change in keratinocytes. Section showing a number of keratinocytes with clear unstained cytoplasm and shrunken nuclei. This pattern must not be confused with Paget's disease. H & E × 240

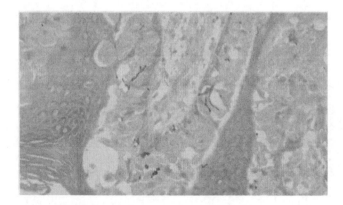

Figure 17.11 Paget's disease of the nipple. A section stained with silver to show black melanin granules in some of the large Paget cells and dendritic melanocytes amongst the cells. Masson-Fontana × 240

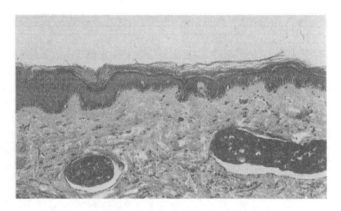

Figure 17.12 Inflammatory carcinoma of the breast. A section of mammary skin from a woman who had a large inflammatory carcinoma of the breast. As shown in this photomicrograph, the typical histological feature is extensive permeation of lymphatics by carcinoma cells. H & E × 96

References

1. Ashikari, R., Park, K., Huvos, A. G. and Urban, J. A. (1970). Paget's disease of the breast. *Cancer*, **26**, 680–685

2. Nance, F. C., DeLoach, D. H., Welsh, R. A. and Becker, W. F. (1970). Paget's disease of the breast. *Ann. Surg.*, **171**, 864–874

3. Paone, J. F. and Baker, R. R. (1981). Pathogenesis and treatment of Paget's disease of the breast. *Cancer*, **48**, 825–829

4. Maor, M. (1979). Significance of eczema in Paget's disease of the breast. *Eur. J. Cancer*, **15**, 35–38

5. Stocks, L. H. and Simmons Patterson, F M . (1976). Inflammatory carcinoma of the breast. *Surg. Gynecol. Obstet.*, **143**, 885–889

6. Lucas, F. V. and Perez-Mesa, C. (1978). Inflammatory carcinoma of the breast. *Cancer*, **41**, 1595–1605

7. Anderson, J. M. (1980). Inflammatory carcinomas of the breast. *Ann. R. Coll. Surg. Engl.*, **62**, 195–199

The most reliable and consistent prognostic factor in mammary carcinoma is the presence or absence of axillary lymph node metastases. However, about one third of patients with negative nodes die from metastatic disease and conversely one third to one half with positive nodes remain alive and well at five years. Therefore, in an attempt to provide more prognostic information various other features, including pathological parameters, have been evaluated over the years. The pathological features which, at one time or another, have been considered to be of possible prognostic significance include tumour type, tumour grade, tumour size, the presence, amount and pattern of the *in situ* component, the shape of the tumour edge, the structure of the stroma, including the degree of stromal elastosis, the presence or absence of necrosis, and the presence or absence of venous and lymphatic invasion. Other features of possible prognostic significance considered. by many to represent a host defence reaction include the intensity and composition of the lymphoplasmacytic cell reaction around and within the tumour, and reactive changes in regional lymph nodes. The significant aspects of metastatic deposits in regional nodes will be considered in the next chapter. Features such as the site of the tumour within the breast, multicentricity and direct involvement of surrounding structures will not be considered here. Of the numerous features of primary mammary carcinoma which have been thought to be possible prognostic indicators, some have been substantiated by multiple studies, but many others have not been shown to be consistently correlated with prognosis. Furthermore, some appear to have limited validity and are not significant in all stages of the disease. Nearly all the prognostic indicators suffer from two major disadvantages: firstly, although many are effective in delineating small groups of patients with either a better or worse prognosis than average, the majority of patients fall into an intermediate category with a very heterogeneous pattern of behaviour; secondly, most of the histological parameters are based on purely subjective assessment and there is often considerable disagreement between observers. The value of various histological features as prognostic indicators has been discussed in several recent reviews[1-4].

The prognostic significance of different tumour types has been considered in the relevant chapters. The most important distinction is between *in situ* and infiltrating carcinoma, but only about 5 to 10% of patients present with pure *in situ* tumours, although the incidence is higher in screening clinics. Other special types of mammary carcinoma with a relatively favourable prognosis include medullary carcinoma with lymphoid stroma, mucoid, tubular, papillary, adenoid cystic and secretory carcinoma. These special types of infiltrating carcinoma together account for up to 10% of all mammary carcinomas, and it is important to realise that the good prognosis associated with these tumours applies only when strict criteria are used in their diagnosis and only when the tumours are pure and not mixed with other more common types of infiltrating carcinoma. These factors may explain some of the discrepancies noted by different observers relating to the prognosis associated with special types of carcinoma.

Although not a histological type of mammary carcinoma, this would appear to be the most appropriate point to consider the concept of minimal carcinoma. This term was originally used to designate *in situ* carcinomas and small infiltrating tumours up to 0.5 cm in maximum dimension. The term has since been extended to include tumours up to 1.0 cm and larger tumours of favourable prognostic types[1,3]. It is also important that the term minimal carcinoma should only be applied to tumours with no associated lymph node metastases. Indeed the use of this term, which includes several different types of tumour, with different patterns of behaviour, is of debatable value. In this context it should also be mentioned that tumour size in general is itself related to prognosis. Although a consistent relationship cannot always be demonstrated, it is well recognized that on the whole prognosis becomes less favourable with increasing tumour size[1-6].

Between 70 and 75% of mammary carcinomas consist of infiltrating duct carcinomas 'not otherwise specified' (NOS) or 'without special features'. The significance of the histological grade in infiltrating duct carcinomas has already been discussed in Chapter 12. Nuclear grading, which is based entirely on the appearance of the nuclei, notably pleomorphism and the number of mitotic figures, and does not take into account the growth pattern of the tumour, can be applied to all types of mammary carcinoma. This system also separates tumours into three categories of differentiation.

The differences in the appearance of the infiltrating edge of mammary carcinomas and variations in the stromal pattern have been illustrated in Chapters 12 and 13. Whilst most tumours display an infiltrating border around all or part of their edge, some have a rounded pushing outline and this has been found to be associated with a more favourable prognosis in several reported series. However, other studies have not confirmed this and indeed sometimes the reverse has been found[3,4].

The amount of elastic tissue within the stroma of a carcinoma has also been considered to be of prognostic significance[7,8]. Elastic tissue is normally present in the breast around ducts and in the walls of vessels and is often increased in carcinomas (Figure 18.1). Large

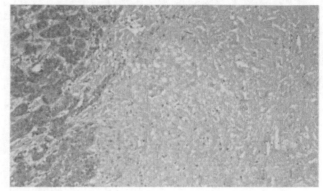

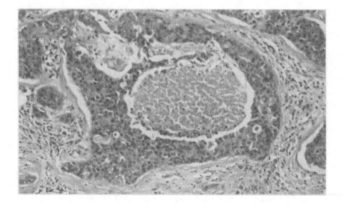

Figure 18.1 Prominent periductal elastosis in carcinoma of the breast. Section prepared from the central part of an infiltrating duct carcinoma with productive fibrosis ['scirrhous' carcinoma]. Thick, black-stained collars of elastic fibres surround many of the ducts. Verhoeff's elastic stain/van Gieson × 24

Figure 18.2 Infarct-like necrosis in infiltrating mammary carcinoma. Surviving, viable tumour can be seen on the left of this photomicrograph, but most of the field is occupied by a large area of coagulative necrosis. Compare with Figure 18.3. H & E × 96

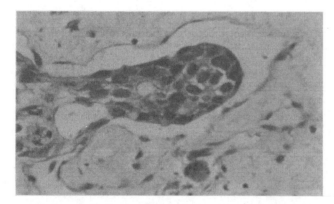

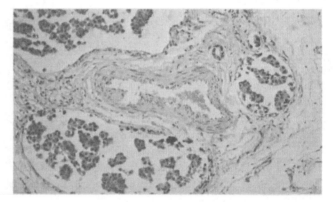

Figure 18.3 Comedo-like necrosis in infiltrating mammary carcinoma. This type is characterized by a circumscribed area of coagulative necrosis, tending to be circular in outline and situated centrally within a relatively small mass of tumour cells. Comedo-like necrosis is seen typically in one variety of intraduct carcinoma ['comedo carcinoma'] but it also occurs in invasive carcinoma and in metastatic breast cancer. H & E × 96

Figure 18.4 Invasion of lymphatic vessels by mammary carcinoma. The artery in the centre of the field is surrounded by widely-dilated lymphatic vessels containing numerous clumps of carcinoma cells. H & E × 96

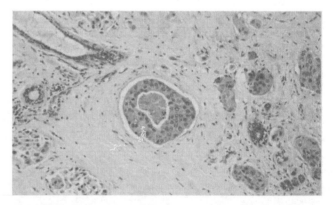

Figure 18.5 Retrograde lymphatic invasion of oedematous limb by carcinoma of the breast. The patient had a radical mastectomy and post-operative radiotherapy for mammary carcinoma. She developed severe lymphoedema of the ipsilateral upper limb, and two years later dermal nodules appeared in the arm. This section was prepared from a biopsy of one nodule. It shows a dilated lymphatic containing a clump of carcinoma cells. The endothelial lining of the vessel is clearly seen. H & E × 240

Figure 18.6 Spurious lymphatic invasion in mammary carcinoma. The mass of carcinoma cells near the centre of the field is lying in a space which suggests a lymphatic vessel on cursory examination. However, critical study shows that there is no endothelial lining to the space, and in other areas clusters of cells and individual cells can be seen to have shrunk away from the surrounding stroma. The appearance is judged to be an artefact of tissue fixation and processing, and not to represent true lymphatic invasion. H & E × 96

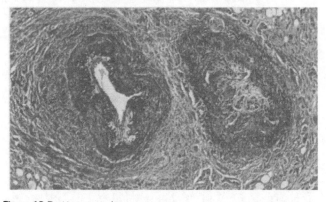

Figure 18.7 Vascular invasion by mammary carcinoma. Section of an infiltrating duct carcinoma of the breast, showing two blood vessels cut transversely. The vessel on the left is an artery: the other is a vein with its lumen occluded by small groups of tumour cells in a fibroblastic stroma. Verhoeff's elastic stain/van Gieson   × 96

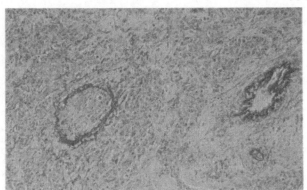

Figure 18.8 Vascular invasion by mammary carcinoma. In this cellular carcinoma, vascular invasion was difficult to detect in haematoxylin and eosin stained preparations. The section illustrated here has been stained for elastic and shows, on the left, a small vein whose lumen is completely filled by tumour cells. An artery is seen on the extreme right. Orcein elastic stain/light green. × 96

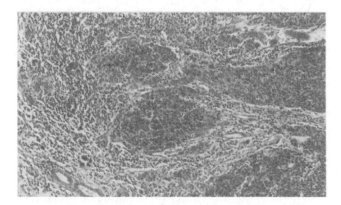

Figure 18.9 Mammary carcinoma with abundant lymphoid stromal infiltrate. This section shows the edge of an infiltrating carcinoma of the breast. The stroma contains a large number of lymphoid cells. At higher magnification, both lymphocytes and plasmacytes could be identified, and there were some large pyroninophilic cells [immunoblasts]. Compare with Figure 18.8. H & E × 96

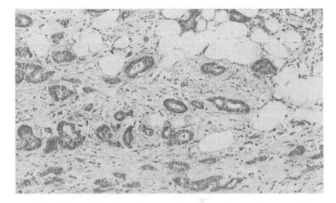

Figure 18.10 Mammary carcinoma with sparse stromal infiltrate. This infiltrating breast cancer shows prominent tubular differentiation. There is a rather loose fibroblastic stroma which contains a few, widely-scattered lymphocytes. Compare with Figure 18.7.   H & E × 96

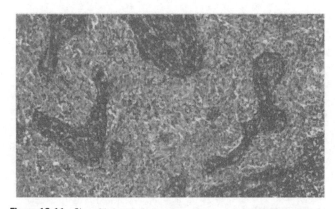

Figure 18.11 Sinus histiocytosis in axillary lymph node. An axillary lymph node from a patient with mammary carcinoma. The sinuses are markedly distended by confluent masses of histiocytes which are relatively large and palely-staining compared with the darkly-staining lymphocytes of the attenuated medullary lymphoid cords.   H & E × 96

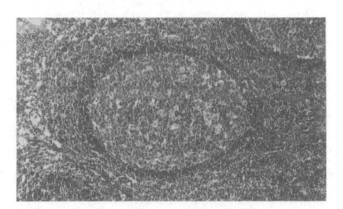

Figure 18.12 Reactive hyperplasia of axillary lymph node. Section of an axillary lymph node from a patient with mammary carcinoma. It showed no sinus histiocytosis, but there are many reaction centres such as the one illustrated here. The centre is surrounded by a peripheral zone of small, darkly-stained lymphocytes. The centre itself comprises a mixture of centroblasts, centrocytes, dendritic reticulum cells, and scattered, vacuolated macrophages; the last-named produce the 'starry-sky' pattern.   H & E × 96

deposits of elastic fibres may also be present elsewhere in the stroma, but whether or not these latter deposits represent remnants of ducts which have been engulfed by the tumour is uncertain. In addition more delicate elastic fibrils are occasionally found. Various reports in the literature correlating the amount of elastic fibres with prognosis are not necessarily comparable, as different workers have not always studied identical patterns of elastic fibre deposition. This may account to some extent for disagreements as to the prognostic significance of elastosis[9]. However, several studies have shown that tumours with a large amount of elastic fibres are associated with a more favourable prognosis than those containing little or none[7,8].

Recently emphasis has been placed on the importance of tumour necrosis as a prognostic indicator[3,5]. Necrosis within duct carcinoma *in situ* is common, but areas of necrosis are not so frequently seen within infiltrating tumours (Figures 18.2 and 18.3). The presence of necrosis in the infiltrating component appears to be associated with a poor prognosis, and the relative amount of necrosis is also significant[5].

Invasion of both lymphatics and blood vessels can sometimes be identified within and around mammary carcinomas. When lymphatic invasion is seen (Figure 18.4), the regional nodes are usually found to contain metastatic tumour. However, the presence of lymphatic invasion in the absence of nodal involvement is important and in two recent studies was found to be the most significant prognostic indicator in small infiltrating tumours without lymph node metastases[10,11]. Artefactual shrinkage of tumour cells from the surrounding stroma must not be confused with true lymphatic invasion (compare Figures 18.5 and 18.6). The wide variation reported in the literature of the incidence of lymphatic involvement (8–38%) may be due to difficulties in recognizing true lymphatic invasion[12]. The presence of blood vessel invasion, usually venous, is also associated with a poor prognosis. In several studies this has been found to be of most significance in patients with stage 2 disease[13,14]. Unfortunately, there is also considerable observer variation in the identification of blood vessel invasion, the reported incidence ranging from 4 to 52%[14]. This discrepancy is again probably due to difficulties of interpretation. Whilst venous invasion can sometimes be identified in routine sections stained with haematoxylin and eosin, elastic stains may be needed to outline the vessel walls (Figures 18.7 and 18.8); even then distinction between veins and ducts can be difficult.

The number of lymphocytes and plasma cells within and around carcinomas varies considerably. A dense cellular reaction is characteristic of medullary carcinoma with lymphoid stroma but a moderately heavy reaction may be seen in other types of carcinoma, and the density can vary from that shown in Figure 18.9 to the minimal infiltrate seen in Figure 18.10. It has long been considered that large numbers of lymphocytes and plasmacytes are indicative of a host defence reaction, and, therefore, their presence indicates a good prognosis. There have been several studies supporting this contention[1,3,4,15]. However, the association has not been universally accepted and indeed some workers claim that a heavy cellular reaction is more often seen around poorly differentiated carcinomas and those with large areas of necrosis, and is therefore associated with a poor prognosis[5,13,16]. In one study, where no overall correlation was found, a significant association was noted between increased cellular reaction and a more favourable prognosis when only poorly differentiated

tumours were considered[16].

Reactive changes within regional lymph nodes have also been regarded as indicative of a host defence reaction and have been correlated with prognosis by several authorities. Again there is no complete agreement but, in general, the presence of sinus histiocytosis (Figure 18.11) in tumour-free axillary nodes has been found to correlate with a good prognosis[1,3,4,17]. It has been suggested that some of the discrepancies relating the association of sinus histiocytosis to prognosis may be due to failure to distinguish 'true' sinus histiocytosis, composed of homogeneous syncytial-like sheets of histiocytes, from a 'degenerative' form where the histiocytes are less compact and are mixed with different cell types[17,18]. Other patterns of lymph node reaction have also been examined but the data here are more limited. The presence of germinal centre activity (Figure 18.12) and a lymphocyte-depleted pattern have both been reported to be of poor prognostic significance[1,3,4,19].

Because of the rather subjective nature of the assessment of most histological features of possible prognostic significance, attempts have been made to use quantitative microscopy in their evaluation[4]. Employing such methods Baak *et al.*[20] analysed several factors including the cellularity index, the mitotic activity index, nuclear measurements and assessment of the nuclear/cytoplasmic ratio.

Although all the features discussed here have been found to have individual prognostic significance, in some centres it has been noted that a combination of the various factors is of more significance than if they are considered individually. With an increase in the number of factors there is a cumulative effect on prognostic prediction[6,21]. However, in general such prognostic indices have not proved to be reproducible.

In future, classification of mammary carcinoma and the evaluation of prognostic features may be based on the identification of tumour products and tumour antigens[2]. The development of immunohistochemical techniques and the use of monoclonal antibodies for detecting tumour markers may well allow for a more objective evaluation.

References

1. McDivitt, R. W. (1978). Breast Carcinoma. *Hum. Pathol.*, **9**, 3–21

2. Rosen, P. P. (1979). The pathological classification of human mammary carcinoma: past, present and future. *Ann. Clin. Lab. Sci.* **9**, 144–156

3. Hutter, R. V. P. (1980). The influence of pathologic factors on breast cancer management. *Cancer*, **46**, 961–976

4. Sharkey, F. E. (1982). Biological meaning of stage and grade in human breast cancer: review and hypothesis. *Breast Cancer Res. Treat.* **2**, 299–322

5. Fisher, E. R., Redmond, C. and Fisher, B. (1980). Pathologic findings from the National Surgical Adjuvant Breast Project (protocol No. 4) VI. Discriminants for five-year treatment failure. *Cancer*, **46**, 908–918

6. Haybittle, J. L., Blamey, R. W., Elston, C. W., Johnson, J., Doyle, P. J., Campbell, F. C., Nicholson, R. I. and Griffiths, K. (1982). A prognostic index in primary breast cancer. *Br. J. Cancer.* **45**, 361–366

7. Shivas, A. A. and Douglas, J. G. (1972). The prognostic significance of elastosis in breast carcinoma. *J. R. Coll. Surg. Edin.*, **17**, 315–320

8. Wallgren, A., Silfversward, C. and Eklund, G. (1976). Prognostic factors in mammary carcinoma. *Acta Radiol.* **15**, 1–16

9. Robertson, A. J., Brown, R. A., Cree, I. A., MacGillivray, J. B., Slidders, W. and Swanson Beck, J. (1981). Prognostic value of measurement of elastosis in breast carcinoma. *J. Clin. Pathol.* **34**, 738–743

10. Rosen, P. P., Saigo, P. E., Braun, D. W. Jr., Weathers, E. and DePalo A. (1981). Predictors of recurrence in Stage I (T1NoMo) breast carcinoma. *Ann. Surg.* **193**, 15–25

11. Roses, D. F., Bell, D. A., Flotte, T. J., Taylor, R., Ratech, H. and Dubin, N. (1982). Pathologic predictors of recurrence in Stage I (T1NoMo) breast cancer. *Am. J. Clin. Pathol.* **78**, 817–820

12. Gilchrist, K. W., Gould, V. E., Hirschl, S., Imbriglia, J. E., Patchefsky, A. S., Penner, D. W., Pickren, J., Schwartz, I. S., Wheeler, J. E., Barnes, J. M. and Mansour, E. G. (1982). Interobserver variation in the identification of breast carcinoma in intramammary lymphatics. *Hum. Pathol.* **13**, 170–2

13. Rosen, P. P., Saigo, P. E., Braun, D. W., Weathers, E. and Kinne, D. W. (1981). Prognosis in Stage II ($T_1N_1M_0$) breast cancer. *Ann. Surg.* **194**, 576–584

14. Weigand, R. A., Isenberg, W. M., Russo, J., Brennan, M. J., Rich, M. A. and associates. (1982). Blood vessel invasion and axillary lymph node involvement as prognostic indicators for human breast cancer. *Cancer,* **50**, 962–969

15. Underwood, J. C. E. (1974). Lymphorecticular infiltration in human tumours: prognostic and biological implications: a review. *Br. J. Cancer,* **30**, 538–548

16. Elston, C. W., Gresham, G. A., Rao, G. S., Zebro, T., Haybittle, J. L., Houghton, J. and Kearney, G. (1982). The cancer research campaign (King's/Cambridge) trial for early breast cancer: clinico-pathological aspects. *Br. J. Cancer.* **45**, 655–669

17. Fisher, E. R., Kotwal, N., Hermann, C., and Fisher, B. (1983). Types of tumor lymphoid response and sinus histiocytosis. *Arch. Pathol. Lab. Med.,* **107**, 222–227

18. Hartveit, F. (1982). The sinus reaction in the axillary nodes in breast cancer related to tumour size and nodal state. *Histopathology,* **6**, 753–764

19. Brynes, R. K., Hunter, R. L. and Vellios, F. (1983). Immunomorphologic changes in regional lymph nodes associated with cancer. *Arch. Pathol. Lab. Med.,* **107**, 217–221

20. Baak, J. P. A., Kurver, P. H. J., De Snoo-Niewlaat, A. J. E., De Graef, S., Makkink, B. and Boon, M. E. (1982). Prognostic indicators in breast cancer – morphometric methods. *Histopathology,* **6**, 327–339

21. Nealon, T. F. Jr., Nkongho, A., Grossi, C. E., Ward, R., Nealon C. and Gillooley, J. F. (1981). Treatment of early cancer of the breast ($T_1N_0M_0$ and $T_2N_0M_0$) on the basis of histologic characteristics. *Surgery,* **89**, 279–289

The prognostic significance of axillary lymph node metastases in carcinoma of the breast is well known, and their presence or absence is the most important single prognostic indicator. As clinical assessment of axillary nodal status gives rise to about a 30% false positive and a 30% false negative rate, histological examination is essential for accurate evaluation.

There are also certain features of involved axillary nodes which give further prognostic information. These are discussed in the review articles mentioned in the previous chapter[1-3]. For some time it has been stressed that patients with three or fewer involved nodes have a considerably better prognosis than those with four or more positive nodes. However, more recently it has been shown that there is a roughly linear correlation between the overall number of positive nodes and the recurrence and survival rates[4].

In many laboratories axillary lymph nodes are dissected into three groups, the low or 'level 1' nodes, below and lateral to the pectoralis minor muscle, the middle or 'level 2' nodes behind the muscle, and the high or 'level 3' nodes above and medial to the edge of pectoralis minor. Survival rates can also be related to the level of nodes containing metastases. Patients with nodes in only level 1 do better than those with nodes in level 2, and patients with nodes in level 3 have a very poor prognosis. There is controversy as to whether the level of node involvement is in fact as important as the total number of involved nodes[1-3]. However, since with increasing numbers of involved nodes there is a greater chance of involvement of levels 2 and 3 it appears that both may be merely different ways of measuring the overall degree of nodal involvement. Although metastases generally progress in an orderly fashion from level 1 through level 2 to level 3, discontinuous or 'skip' metastases occur in about 3% of patients with positive nodes[5].

The histological identification of lymph node metastases usually presents no problem to the pathologist. However, metastases are occasionally missed, either by being overlooked because they are of small size or because they have an unusual microscopic pattern which is misinterpreted. There have been several studies indicating that routine methods of examining lymph nodes miss about 20–30% of small metastatic lesions, although it has generally been found that such small metastases (less than 2 mm maximal diameter) do not appear to affect survival[1-3]. However, there is a divergence of opinion both in regard to the dimension of the critical size and as to the prognostic significance of these micrometastases. For example, Fisher et al.[6] found the critical size to be 1.3 mm rather than 2 mm. Furthermore, Rosen et al.[7] in a study of the significance of single lymph node metastases found that the survival curves in their series varied with the size of the primary carcinoma. When the primary tumours were 2 cm or less, the presence of micrometastases had no deleterious effect on prognosis during the first 6 years of follow-up, but at 12 years the survival rates for patients with micro- and macrometastases were nearly identical. On the other hand, when the patients had mammary carcinomas measuring 2.1–5 cm, those with a single micrometastasis showed survival curves similar to those with negative nodes throughout the course of follow-up.

Most metastases commence in the peripheral sinus of the node, and therefore careful scrutiny of this region is essential for the detection of small lesions such as is shown in Figure 19.1. Unusual patterns of metastatic involvement are sometimes seen, particularly with infiltrating lobular carcinoma. Metastatic tumour confined to the sinusoids (Figure 19.2) may on initial examination be mistaken for sinus histiocytosis, but careful scrutiny of the infiltrating cells reveals their true nature. In Figure 19.3, although most of the node is replaced by tumour, the germinal centres are spared and again this could be confused with a reactive pattern. Sometimes the picture is reversed and nodules of malignant cells can be mistaken for germinal centres. In Figures 19.4–19.6, the whole node is replaced by metastatic tumour, a picture closely resembling a malignant lymphoma. In some nodal deposits a large amount of fibrous stroma is produced. Another unusual pattern is shown in Figure 19.7. Although this appearance should produce no diagnostic difficulty, it strongly resembles *in situ* duct carcinoma. Of course the presence of such a lesion within a lymph node precludes this diagnosis, but its occurrence indicates that such a pattern does not always represent *in situ* carcinoma when seen within the breast, since it can clearly develop in infiltrating mammary carcinoma.

In Figure 19.8 metastatic tumour is seen extending through the capsule of the node. The presence of extranodal extension has been found to be associated with a poor prognosis[1-3]. It is usually seen when the axilla is heavily involved but is of particular significance in patients with three or fewer involved axillary nodes[8]. Extension of the metastasis through the capsule should be distinguished from the presence of tumour cells within the capsule as this latter appearance does not necessarily indicate a poor prognosis. Tumour cells are sometimes seen in perinodal vessels (veins and lymphatics) and indicate a poor prognosis (Figure 19.9 and 19.10). Hartveit[9] has found that the presence of malignant cells within the efferent vessels (either veins or lymphatics) of a node is associated with a particularly poor prognosis, probably related to tertiary spread. Efferent vascular spread is usually seen in nodes already largely replaced by metastatic tumour. These lymphatics will only be demonstrated if the node is sectioned

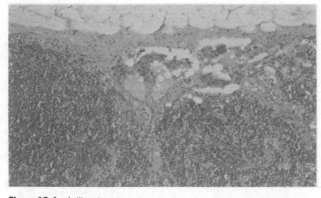

Figure 19.1 Axillary lymph node: minute deposit of secondary carcinoma in peripheral sinus. Perinodal adipose tissue and the capsule are situated in the upper part of the field. The peripheral sinus is slightly dilated; it contains some eosinophilic proteinaceous coagulum and a few small clusters of carcinoma cells.   H & E × 96

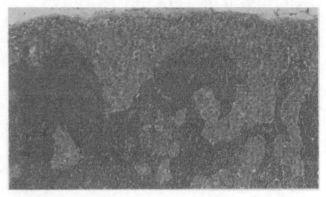

Figure 19.2 Axillary lymph node: secondary carcinoma permeating sinusoids. The peripheral sinus is expanded by a mass of cohesive carcinoma cells, and from the periphery columns of cells have extended into the sinusoids passing into the deeper part of the node. The sinusoids are sharply delineated from the surrounding, small, darkly-stained lymphocytes of the pulp.   H & E × 96

Figure 19.3 Axillary lymph node: secondary lobular carcinoma of the breast. In this node, the tumour cells display a diffuse pattern of infiltration, with minimal supporting stroma. Much of the normal architecture of the node has been effaced, but lymphoid follicles, such as the one on the left of the field, have survived.   H & E × 96

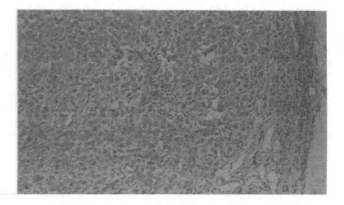

Figure 19.4 Axillary lymph node: total replacement by secondary carcinoma. The capsule is present on the extreme right. Apart from a very few scattered lymphocytes, all the normal lymph node structure has been destroyed and replaced by a mass of carcinoma cells.   H & E × 96

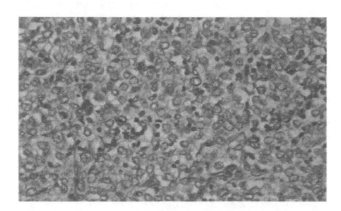

Figure 19.5 Axillary lymph node: secondary lobular carinoma of the breast. High power view of a diffusely infiltrating secondary carcinoma in an axillary lymph node. The tumour cells have vesicular nuclei and ill-defined boundaries. There is no obvious supporting stroma. A few lymphocytes are intermingled. A secondary neoplasm with this pattern may be mistaken for a malignant lymphoma, of histiocytic or centroblastic type.   H & E × 240

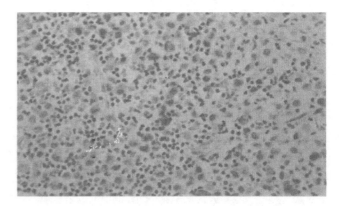

Figure 19.6 Axillary lymph node: secondary carcinoma of the breast. Another section of the lymph node illustrated in Figure 19.5. Many of the tumour cells contain PAS-positive, diastase resistant mucin, stained red.   PAS after diastase digestion × 240

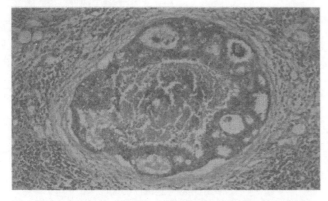

Figure 19.7 Axillary lymph node: secondary carcinoma displaying cribriform pattern and comedo-type necrosis. Section of an axillary lymph node from a 55-year-old woman with intraduct and infiltrating carcinoma of the breast. The secondary deposit shown here is surrounded by a zone of fibrosis, and displays a cribriform pattern, central necrosis and focal calcification. The similarity to *in situ* duct carcinoma, as seen in primary breast cancer, is evident. H & E × 96

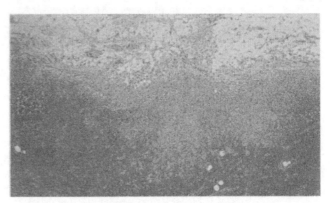

Figure 19.8 Axillary lymph node: extension of secondary carcinoma into perinodal tissues. Secondary carcinoma has extended from the peripheral sinus into the substance of the lymph node, and has also penetrated the capsule to invade the perinodal fat. H & E × 24

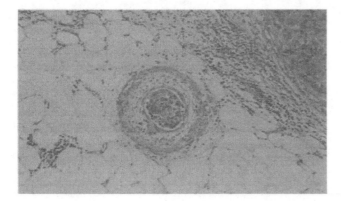

Figure 19.9. Axillary lymph node: carcinoma cells within extranodal vein. Part of the node, containing secondary carcinoma, is seen in the top right-hand corner of the field. At the centre of the photograph, there is a small vein lying in the perinodal adipose tissue. The intima of the vessel is thickened and its lumen is plugged with carcinoma cells. H & E × 96

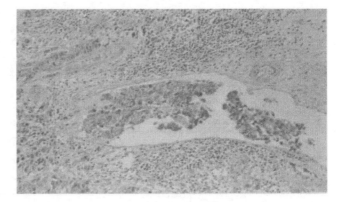

Figure 19.10 Axillary lymph node: secondary carcinoma within an efferent lymphatic vessel. This section shows part of the hilar region of a lymph node from a patient with an infiltrating duct carcinoma of the breast. The dilated vessel running transversely across the field is an efferent lymphatic containing large, irregularly-shaped clumps of secondary carcinoma cells. H & E × 96

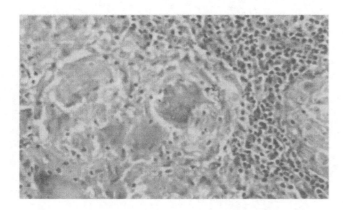

Figure 19.11 Axillary lymph node: tuberculoid granuloma associated with mammary carcinoma. An axillary lymph node from a radical mastectomy specimen. The patient had an infiltrating duct carcinoma of the breast. No metastatic tumour was present in this lymph node, but the section shows a non-caseating tuberculoid granuloma, composed of epithelioid cells and many multinucleated giant cells. H & E × 240

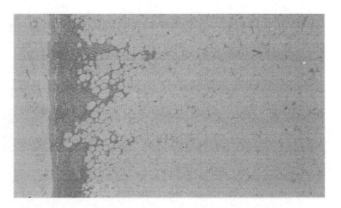

Figure 19.12 Adipose tissue in axillary lymph node of axilla. Photomicrograph of a large axillary lymph node, judged to be probably involved by secondary carcinoma on clinical examination. The capsule and some perinodal fat are seen on the left. Beneath the capsule, there is a peripheral sinus and a narrow zone of lymphoid tissue. The rest of the node is occupied by mature adipose tissue. There is no secondary tumour. H & E × 24

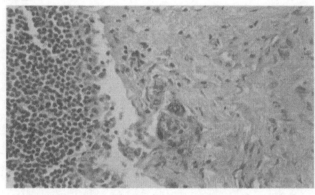

Figure 19.13 Axillary lymph node: naevus cells in capsule. An axillary lymph node from a woman with carcinoma of the breast. The thickened capsule occupies the right half of the field; within it there is a small cluster of cells containing brown pigment which gave the staining reactions for melanin. In the left half of the photograph are the peripheral sinus and subjacent lymphoid tissue.   H & E × 240

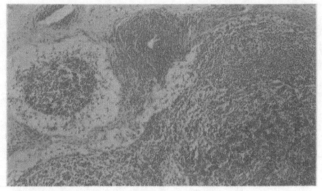

Figure 19.14 Axillary lymph node: naevus cells in capsule. Section of an axillary lymph node from a radical mastectomy specimen. Part of the capsule is seen at the top of the field, and the subjacent peripheral sinus is dilated. Within the capsule there is a large cluster of naevus cells. The cells have small, regular nuclei, and have no resemblance to the larger, pleomorphic cells of the mammary carcinoma.   H & E × 96

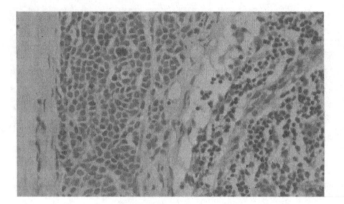

Figure 19.15 Axillary lymph node: naevus cells in capsule. In the left half of the field, there is a large, elongated cluster of naevus cells within the capsule. Note the regular size, shape and staining properties of the naevus cells. Mitotic figures are absent.   H & E × 240

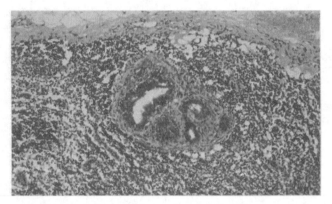

Figure 19.16 Axillary lymph node: benign epithelial inclusions. The lymph node capsule is seen at the edge of the field. In the central part of the photograph, there is a cluster of epithelial tubules with a supporting connective tissue stroma. The tubules display a double cell layer. This is an example of epithelial heterotopia, a condition which is uncommon in axillary lymph nodes.   H & E × 96

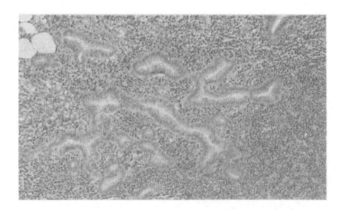

Figure 19.17 Axillary lymph node: benign epithelial inclusions. In this example, the heterotopic epithelium is arranged as narrow, branching tubules, without a conspicuous supporting stroma. Special stains (PAS, trichrome and reticulin preparations) show all the tubules to be surrounded by regular basement membranes. The epithelial cells are regular in size, shape and staining properties, and mitotic figures are absent.   H & E × 96

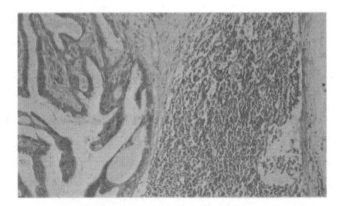

Figure 19.18 Axillary lymph node: benign epithelial inclusions. The capsule, peripheral sinus and subjacent lymphoid tissue occupy the right half of the field. On the left, there is heterotopic epithelium with surrounding connective tissue. The epithelial structures display cyst formation, papillary ingrowths and pink cell metaplasia.   H & E × 96

through the hilum, so it is not always practicable to demonstrate this feature.

Various reactive changes have been described in lymph nodes draining malignant tumours. The significance of sinus histiocytosis and germinal centre activity has already been discussed in Chapter 18, on prognostic features. Another well recognized feature is the presence of giant cell granulomas (Figure 19.11); their significance is not known but they must be distinguished from metastatic deposits.

Fibrosis of lymph node sinusoids is not uncommon, particularly in older patients, and calcium may be deposited in the fibrous tissue. Thus calcification within the axillary nodes, occasionally detected on mammography, does not necessarily indicate the presence of metastatic tumour. Another change, more usually seen in elderly women, is illustrated in Figure 19.12. Fatty replacement of lymph nodes is particularly common in obese women and sometimes the nodes appear to be markedly enlarged on clinical examination.

The occurrence of naevus cell nests within lymph nodes is well recognized and although described in lymph nodes from various sites is most often seen in the axillary nodes[10-12]. The naevus cells are present in the capsule of the node (Figures 19.13–19.15) and may extend into the node within trabeculae but are not seen within the sinusoids or parenchyma. The only importance of this phenomenon is its possible confusion with secondary tumour. Similarly the presence of benign mammary tissue within lymph nodes, a rare but well-established occurrence, must be distinguished from metastatic involvement[13]. These benign glandular inclusions may resemble normal mammary structures but can also show benign pathological changes similar to those seen in the breast (Figures 19.16–19.18). A case of papillary carcinoma apparently arising from ectopic breast tissue in an axillary lymph node has also been reported[14].

Lymph nodes are occasionally found within the anatomical confines of the breast and may present as a breast lump. These intramammary lymph nodes may be involved in a variety of non-specific and specific reactive and inflammatory processes, as mentioned in Chapter 4, and infarction of an intramammary node has been seen following needle aspiration biopsy[15]. Additionally, they may be involved by metastatic tumour. In a recent study of mastectomy specimens from patients with mammary carcinoma, Egan and McSweeney[16] found intramammary nodes in 28% of breasts and 10% contained metastatic deposits. Lymph nodes low in the axillary tail of the breast also sometimes present as a breast mass. Histologically, reactive changes may be present but frequently no significant abnormality is seen. Sometimes such nodes become apparent in women who have recently lost weight.

References

1. McDivitt, R. W. (1978). Breast carcinoma. *Hum. Pathol.,* **9**, 3–21

2. Hutter, R. V.P. (1980). The influence of pathologic factors on breast cancer management. *Cancer,* **46**, 961–976

3. Sharkey, F. E. (1982). Biological meaning of stage and grade in human breast cancer: review and hypothesis. *Breast Cancer Res. Treat.,* **2**, 299–322

4. Nemoto, T., Vana, J., Bedwani, R. N., Baker, H. W., McGregor, F. H. and Murphy, G. P. (1980). Management and survival of breast cancer: results of a national survey by the American College of Surgeons. *Cancer,* **45**, 2917–2924

5. Rosen, P. P., Lesser, M. L., Kinne, D. W. and Beattie, E. J. (1983). Discontinuous or 'skip' metastases in breast carcinoma. Analysis of 1228 axillary dissections. *Ann Surg.,* **197**, 276–293

6. Fisher, E. R., Palekar, A., Rockette, H., Redmond, C. and Fisher, B. (1978). Pathologic findings from the National Surgical Adjuvant Breast Project (protocol No.4). V. Significance of axillary nodal micro and macrometastases. *Cancer,* **42**, 2032–2038

7. Rosen, P. P. Saigo, P. E., Braun, D. W., Weathers, E., Fracchia, A. A. and Kinne, D. W. (1981). Axillary micro- and macrometastases in breast cancer. *Ann. Surg.,* **194**, 585–591

8. Mambo, N. C. and Gallager, H. S. (1977). Carcinoma of the breast. The prognostic significance of extranodal extension of axillary disease. *Cancer,* **39**, 2280–2285

9. Hartveit, F., Skjaerven, R. and Maehle, B. O. (1983). Prognosis in breast cancer patients with tumour cells in the efferent vessels of their axillary nodes. *J. Pathol.,* **139**, 379–382

10. Johnson, W. T. and Helwig, E. B. (1969). Benign nevus cells in the capsule of lymph nodes. *Cancer,* **23**, 747–753

11. Ridolfi, R. L., Rosen, P. P. and Thaler, H (1977). Nevus cell aggregates associated with lymph nodes: estimated frequency and clinical significance. *Cancer,* **39**, 164–171

12. Erlandson, R. A. and Rosen, P. P. (1982) Electron microscopy of a nevus cell aggregate associated with an axillary lymph node. *Cancer,* **49**, 269–272

13. Turner, D. R. and Millis, R. R. (1980). Breast tissue inclusions in axillary lymph nodes. *Histopathology,* **4**, 631–636

14. Walker, A. N. and Fechner, R. E. (1982). Papillary carcinoma arising from ectopic breast tissue in an axillary lymph node. *Diagnosc. Gynecol. Obstet.,* **4**, 141–145

15. Davies, J. D. and Webb, A. J. (1982). Segmental lymph-node infarction after fine-needle aspiration. *J. Clin. Pathol.,* **35**, 855–857

16. Egan, R. L. and McSweeney, M. B. (1983). Intramammary lymph nodes. *Cancer,* **51**, 1838–1842

20

Benign Soft Tissue Tumours and Tumour-like Conditions

Lipoma

Lipoma is probably the most common benign soft-tissue neoplasm of the breast; its gross and microscopic appearance are similar to those of lipomas occurring elsewhere in the body. Occasionally, glandular elements are incorporated within the substance of the tumour, and the term 'adenolipoma' has been applied to such a lesion. Another variant is angiolipoma which microscopically features a rich plexus of capillary blood vessels interspersed between the lipocytes (Figure 20.1).

Angioma

Benign angiomas of the breast are rare, and are usually small; most frequently, an angioma is a coincidental finding in breast tissue removed for some other reason. Rosen and Ridolfi[1] found an incidence of 1.2% of microscopic perilobular haemangiomas in mastectomy specimens performed for mammary carcinoma. Perilobular haemangiomas consist of meshworks of thin-walled, dilated vascular channels situated either within lobules or in the extralobular mammary stroma (Figure 20.2). As emphasized in Chapter 22, any vascular tumour of the breast which is clinically apparent should be suspected of being an angiosarcoma, although this dictum applies only to lesions actually within the breast substance and not to those situated more superficially in the dermis or subcutaneous tissue. Nevertheless, larger vascular tumours with the features of subcutaneous cavernous haemangiomas do occasionally occur within the breast[2]. The lesion illustrated in Figure 20.3 presented clinically as a breast cyst which yielded bloodstained fluid on aspiration and was subsequently excised. In a benign angioma, there is no evidence of pleomorphism or hyperchromasia of the lining endothelial cells, and there are distinct connective-tissue bands between the vascular spaces. There are a few reports of haemangiopericytomas arising within breast tissue[3].

Granular Cell Tumour (Granular Cell Myoblastoma)

The occurrence of granular cell myoblastoma within the breast is relatively uncommon, but nevertheless important because of its possible confusion with carcinoma[4-6]. The lesion may arise either within the breast substance or in the overlying skin. Those lesions within the substance of the breast are the ones most likely to cause diagnostic difficulties. The tumours may be hard, and can be fixed to deep or superficial structures, distorting and even ulcerating the overlying skin. Macroscopically they are usually creamy-white in colour and firm in consistency. Histologically granular cell tumours may be confused with carcinomas, especially during the examination of frozen sections. The neoplasms have a microscopic appearance similar to that of myoblastomas occuring at other sites, being composed of plump cells with rather indistinct cell borders, uniform round central nuclei and eosinophilic granular cytoplasm (Figure 20.4). The cells are arranged in compact nests and cords separated by a fibrous stroma.

Leiomyoma

Leiomyomas rarely occur within the substance of the breast, although they are not uncommon in the region of the nipple (Figures 20.5 and 20.6). At the latter site, they are thought to arise from the erectile muscle of the nipple[7]. Leiomyomas are composed of interlacing bundles of fusiform cells with the typical blunt-ended nuclei as seen in such neoplasms arising elsewhere in the body.

The occurrence of smooth muscle in other benign breast lesions is described by Eusebi et al.[8].

Benign Chondrolipomatous Tumour

Although the presence of cartilage and bone in malignant tumours of the breast is well documented, it is an unusual feature of benign mammary lesions. Apart from the occasional occurrence of bone and cartilage in fibroadenomas and benign phyllodes tumours, both may also be found in the rare mixed tumours of the breast similar to those of salivary glands. In all of these neoplasms, both epithelial and mesenchymal elements are present. However, a few benign tumours reported in the literature have been composed entirely of various stromal elements, including cartilage, bone and fat[9,10]. The benign chondrolipomatous tumour is one of these. It is a rare lesion which comprises a well-demarcated nodule composed of islands of mature hyaline cartilage with intervening fat and fibrous tissue (Figure 20.7). Occasionally glandular elements are incorporated. There is no cellular atypia, mitotic activity or necrosis, and there should be no difficulty in distinguishing chondrolipomas from malignant mammary neoplasms.

Benign Chondro-osseous and Osseous Tumours of the Breast

The breast is an uncommon site for the development of these lesions, which are also composed entirely of mesenchymal elements (Figures 20.8 and 20.9). They are considered to be identical to the benign (pseudo-malignant) osseous tumour of soft tissue seen in other anatomical situations[11,12].

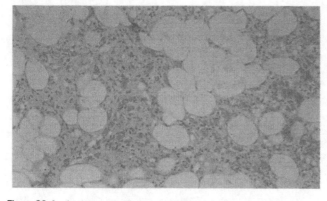

Figure 20.1 Angiolipoma of the breast. Section of a sharply-circumscribed, ovoid, fatty nodule excised from the breast of a 25-year-old woman. Microscopically the lesion is composed of mature lipocytes, and there are areas, as illustrated here, in which capillary blood vessels are very numerous. This is the typical appearance of angiolipoma as seen in other sites.   H & E × 96

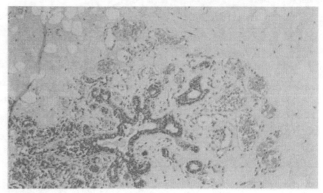

Figure 20.2 Perilobular haemangioma. Sections showing a mammary lobule with a surrounding mantle of thin-walled blood vessels. The lesion was an incidental microscopic finding and was confined to this field. The endothelial cells displayed no pleomorphism, hyperchromasia nor mitotic activity, and there were no uncanalized cellular areas or papillary tufting. H & E × 24

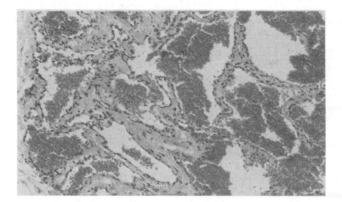

Figure 20.3 Cavernous haemangioma of the breast. Section of a well-circumscribed, deep-red nodule from the breast of a young woman. The lesion comprises wide vascular spaces, with fibrous-tissue walls, lined by single layers of endothelial cells. The endothelium displays no nuclear aberration nor mitotic activity. The thin-walled anastomosing channels of an angiosarcoma are absent, and there is no endothelial tufting, papillary formation nor cellular areas. The patient remains free from recurrence 5 years after simple local excision of the lesion.   H & E × 96

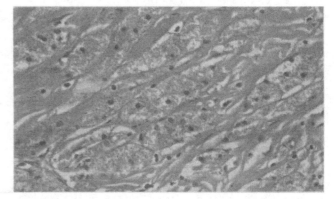
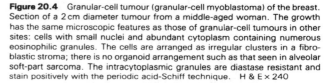

Figure 20.4 Granular-cell tumour (granular-cell myoblastoma) of the breast. Section of a 2 cm diameter tumour from a middle-aged woman. The growth has the same microscopic features as those of granular-cell tumours in other sites: cells with small nuclei and abundant cytoplasm containing numerous eosinophilic granules. The cells are arranged as irregular clusters in a fibroblastic stroma; there is no organoid arrangement such as that seen in alveolar soft-part sarcoma. The intracytoplasmic granules are diastase resistant and stain positively with the periodic acid-Schiff technique.   H & E × 240

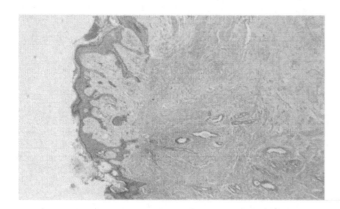

Figure 20.5 Leiomyoma of the nipple. Section of a firm, ill-defined nodule in the nipple, showing interwoven bundles of smooth muscle surrounding and compressing the lactiferous ducts. The epidermis is intact. The lesion is completely unencapsulated.   H & E × 24

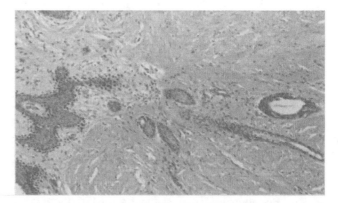

Figure 20.6 Leiomyoma of the nipple. Higher magnification of the lesion illustrated in Figure 20.5. Part of the epidermis is seen on the extreme left. The smooth muscle stains more intensely with eosin than the collagen of the dermis. Mammary ducts have become entrapped by the tumour. The nuclei of the muscle cells are regular in size, shape and staining properties, and there are no mitotic figures.   H & E × 96

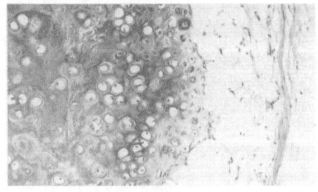

Figure 20.7 Chondrolipoma of the breast. Section of a well-circumscribed spheroidal tumour from the breast of a young woman. The lesion is composed of mature adipose tissue, with multiple nodules of well-differentiated hyaline cartilage. There was no recurrence 6 years after simple excision. H & E × 96

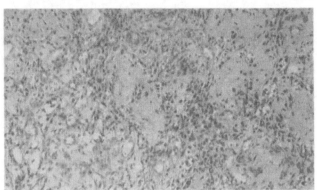

Figure 20.8 Benign (pseudomalignant) osseous tumour of soft parts. Section of a mass, 4 cm in diameter, involving the mammary region of a 13-year-old girl; it was adherent to the underlying chest wall. This photograph shows the central part of the tumour. There is considerable cellular pleomorphism and hyperchromasia. Some osteoid is present, but no well-formed bone trabeculae have developed. H & E × 96

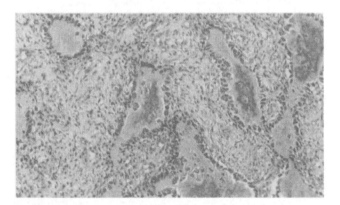

Figure 20.9 Benign (pseudomalignant) osseous tumour of soft parts. From the same lesion as that illustrated in Figure 20.8. This section has been prepared from the periphery of the mass, and shows maturation of the tissue to bone trabeculae with prominent osteoblastic rimming, the 'zone phenomenon'. The patient remained well, without evidence of tumour recurrence, 10 years after simple excision of the lesion. H & E × 96

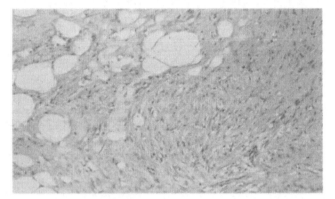

Figure 20.10 Infiltrative fibromatosis (extra-abdominal desmoid tumour) of the breast. Section showing part of an ill-defined stellate mass from the breast of a young woman. The lesion is composed of highly differentiated fibroblasts, with abundant collagen. There are no cytological features indicative of a sarcoma, but the proliferating lesional tissue infiltrates locally and there is no formation of a capsule or pseudocapsule. The photomicrograph shows part of the main bulk of the tumour on the right, with extension into the mammary adipose tissue on the left. H & E × 96

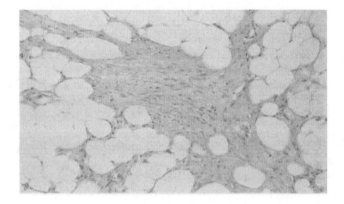

Figure 20.11 Infiltrative fibromatosis of the breast. Another part of the lesion illustrated in Figure 20.10. This section was prepared from tissue situated some distance from the periphery of the main mass, and shows how tentacles of fibrous tissue ramify into the surrounding fat. H & E × 96

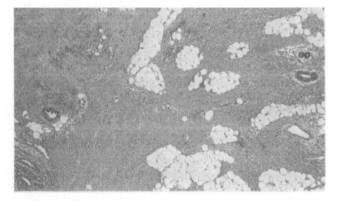

Figure 20.12 Infiltrative fibromatosis of the breast. A section stained by a trichrome technique, collagen being coloured blue. The infiltrating fibrous tissue surrounds and entraps islands of adipose tissue. On the extreme right and left of the field, engulfed mammary ducts can also be seen. Picro-Mallory × 24

Fibromatosis

Infiltrative fibromatosis arising primarily within the substance of the breast is very unusual, although the breast may be secondarily involved by such a lesion developing in adjacent structures such as the pectoral muscle. The gross and histological appearances (Figures 20.10–20.12) and the treatment are the same as those of fibromatosis occurring at other sites[13,14].

Neurofibroma and Neurolemmoma

Nerve sheath tumours of the breast are rare, but are occasionally encountered and are microscopically identical to such tumours arising elsewhere[15].

Miscellaneous Mesenchymal Lesions

A number of very rare and unusual mesenchymal breast lesions, of uncertain nature and behaviour, have been reported. These include 'benign spindle cell' breast tumour[16] and infiltrating myoepithelioma[17].

References

1. Rosen, P. P. and Ridolfi, R. L. (1977). The perilobular hemangioma. A benign microscopic vascular lesion of the breast. *Am. J. Clin. Pathol.,* **68**, 21–23

2. Donnell, R. M., Rosen, P. P., Lieberman, P. H., Kaufman, R. J., Kay, S., Braun, D. W. Jr. and Kinne, D. W. (1981). Angiosarcoma and other vascular tumours of the breast. Pathologic analysis as a guide to prognosis. *Am. J. Surg. Pathol.,* **5**, 629

3. Tavassoli, F. A. and Weiss, S. (1981). Hemangiopericytoma of the breast. *Am. J. Surg. Pathol.,* **5**, 745–752

4. Mulcare, R. (1968). Granular cell myoblastoma of the breast. *Ann. Surg.,* **168**, 262–268

5. Umansky, C. and Bullock, W. K. (1968). Granular cell myoblastoma of the breast. *Ann. Surg.,* **168**, 810–817

6. McCracken, M., Hamal, P. B. and Benson, E. A. (1979). Granular cell myoblastoma of the breast: a report of 2 cases. *Br. J. Surg.,* **66**, 819–821

7. Nascimento, A. G., Karas, M., Rosen, P. P. and Caron, A. G. (1979). Leiomyoma of the nipple. *Am. J. Surg. Pathol.,* **3**, 151–154

8. Eusebi, V., Cunsolo, A., Fedeli, F., Severi, B. and Scarani, P. (1980). Benign smooth muscle cell metaplasia in breast. *Tumori,* **66**, 643–653

9. Dharkar, D. D. and Kraft, J. R. (1981). Benign chondro-lipomatous tumour of the breast. *Postgrad. Med. J.,* **57**, 129–131

10. Kaplan, L. and Walts, A. E. (1977). Benign chondrolipomatous tumor of the human female breast. *Arch. Pathol. Lab. Med.,* **101**, 149–151

11. Ackerman, L. V. (1958). Extra-osseous localized non-neoplastic bone and cartilage formation (so-called myositis ossificans). Clinical and pathological confusion with malignant neoplasms. *J. Bone Joint Surg.,* **40-A**, 279–298

12. Angervall, L., Stener, B., Stener, I. and Ahren, C. (1969). Pseudo-malignant osseous tumour of soft tissue. *J. Bone Joint Surg.,* **51B**, 654–663

13. Ali, M., Fayemi, A. O., Braun, E. V. and Remy, R. (1979). Fibromatosis of the breast. *Am. J. Surg. Pathol.,* **3**, 501–505

14. Gump, F.E., Sternschein, M. J. and Wolff, M. (1981). Fibromatosis of the breast. *Surg. Gynecol. Obstet.,* **153**, 57–60

15. Sherman, J. E. and Smith, J. W. (1981). Neurofibromas of the breast and nipple–areolar area. *Ann. Plast. Surg.,* **7**, 302–307

16. Toker, C., Tang, C.-K., Whitely, J. F., Berkheiser, S. W. and Rachman, R. (1981). Benign spindle cell breast tumor. *Cancer,* **48**, 1615–1622

17. Erlandson, R. A. and Rosen, P. P. (1982). Infiltrating myoepithelioma of the breast. *Am. J. Surg. Pathol.,* **6**, 785–793

Sarcomas – Malignant Cystosarcoma Phyllodes Tumour, Pure Sarcoma, Postmastectomy Lymphangiosarcoma, Radiation-induced Sarcoma, Carcinosarcoma

21

Soft tissue sarcomas of the breast can arise directly from the mammary stroma or may be part of a fibro-epithelial neoplasm. Thus they may be subdivided into two groups according to whether or not a benign epithelial component is associated with the sarcoma.

Malignant Cystosarcoma Phyllodes (Malignant Phyllodes) Tumour

When there is a benign epithelial component the neoplasm is designated malignant cystosarcoma phyllodes tumour or preferably malignant phyllodes tumour. As previously mentioned, the term 'cystosarcoma' is not ideal but is still often used and as long as it is qualified as either benign or malignant the terminology should not lead to any misunderstanding. There is considerable variation in the reported relative incidence of malignant and benign phyllodes tumours; estimates of malignancy have ranged from 8 to 54%[1]. This variation is probably dependent on several factors; the inherent difficulty in distinguishing between the benign and malignant tumours with certainty; the use of differing criteria for the diagnosis of phyllodes tumours; and because some reports are from centres where an unusually high proportion of malignant cases have been referred for consultation[1]. The true rate of malignancy is probably about 20%. As stated earlier in Chapter 7, the term cystosarcoma phyllodes or phyllodes tumour should be reserved for that distinctive type of fibroepithelial neoplasm which possesses the characteristic cellular stroma[2]. Whether phyllodes tumours arise *de novo*, or originate in a pre-existing fibroadenoma, is unclear. Certainly in some tumours, either benign or malignant, areas with the typical microscopic appearance of a conventional fibroadenoma can be found.

The average age of patients with phyllodes tumours is 45 years, somewhat older than that for simple fibroadenomas[1,2]; and in several series the mean age for patients with malignant tumours has been found to be a few years greater than that for patients with benign lesions[2-4]. Malignant lesions are extremely rare under the age of 25 years[5]. An interesting clinical feature of phyllodes tumours is that patients with malignant lesions usually have a longer history than those with benign growths, and, not infrequently, they state that a lump has been present for a long time, but has shown recent rapid increase in size[2,3]. Bilateral phyllodes tumours are rare but have been reported[2,3]. Both benign and malignant variants have been recorded in men[6]. The clinical features vary, and even in patients with benign growths there may be skin ulceration, due simply to the rapid growth of a very large tumour. Axillary node enlargement is common but is almost invariably due to reactive hyperplasia rather than the presence of secondary tumour.

The gross appearance of a phyllodes tumour is similar in both the benign and malignant forms (Figure 21.1), and has been described previously in Chapter 7. Although the average size of benign lesions is usually smaller than that of malignant lesions, benign tumours can be very large, whilst very small tumours occasionally give rise to metastases. On histological examination the basic architecture of a fibroadenoma is apparent, usually with an exaggerated intracanalicular pattern (Figures 21.2 and 21.3) and always with the hypercellular stroma characteristic of these neoplasms (Figures 21.4 and 21.5). Distinction between benign and malignant phyllodes tumours is not always easy and occasionally tumours with a benign histological appearance can run an aggressive clinical course and conversely those with an ominous histological pattern may behave in a benign fashion[2,3]. However, there are various histological features which may be helpful in distinguishing benign from malignant lesions. As microscopic evidence of malignancy may be confined to only a small area of the neoplasm, wide sampling is mandatory. Probably the most important feature indicative of malignancy is increased mitotic activity (Figure 21.6). An average of 3 or more mitotic figures per 10 high power fields is suggestive of malignancy and the presence of 5 or more mitotic figures per 10 high power fields is strongly indicative that the neoplasm will behave in an aggressive fashion. Another feature strongly suggestive of malignancy is marked overgrowth of the stroma relative to the epithelial component as shown in Figure 21.7. Some parts of the tumour may consist entirely of stroma, with no epithelium being apparent.

Blocks prepared from the periphery of a tumour should be examined carefully, as the presence of an infiltrating edge (Figure 21.8) as opposed to a pushing border (Figure 21.9) is also indicative of malignancy, although it is not essential for the diagnosis and indeed the tumour illustrated in Figure 21.9 was malignant. Marked atypia is another feature suggestive of malignancy, but again is not seen in all aggressive tumours. Because of the difficulties in making a definite distinction between benign and malignant tumours some workers include a 'borderline' category in their classification[3,4].

In malignant phyllodes tumours the histological structure of the stroma is usually that of fibrosarcoma (Figures 21.4–6 and 21.8–10), but metaplasia is common and may result in the appearance of fat, and more rarely cartilage, bone, striated muscle and very rarely smooth muscle, or the features of a malignant fibrous histiocytoma may be produced[2-4,7-9]. On other occasions the sarcomatous element is completely undifferentiated (Figure 21.7), and may be difficult to

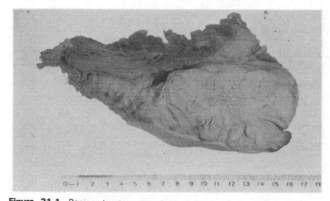

Figure 21.1 Benign (cystosarcoma) phyllodes tumour. Bisected mastectomy specimen showing a large, lobulated, greyish tumour, extending from the skin to the pectoral muscle. The cut surface displays the characteristic clefts

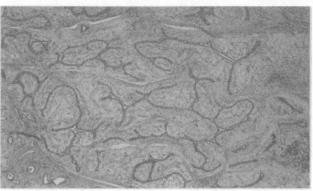

Figure 21.2 Malignant (cystosarcoma) phyllodes tumour. Section at low magnification, showing intracanalicular tubules.   H & E × 24

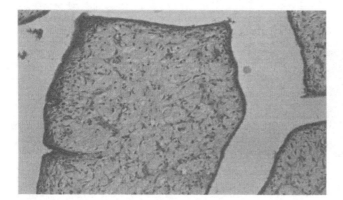

Figure 21.3 Malignant (cystosarcoma) phyllodes tumour. Section shows clefting along epithelial-lined spaces, such clefts may be apparent macroscopically. The mesenchymal component is myxoid and features some spheroidal cells with peripheral nuclei and vacuolated cytoplasm, probably lipoblasts. In other areas the stroma was more cellular and had become frankly sarcomatous. From the same tumour as that illustrated in Figure 21.2. H & E × 96

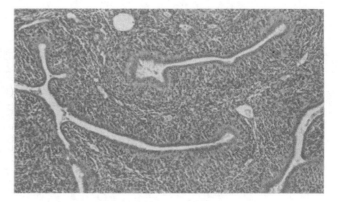

Figure 21.4 Malignant (cystosarcoma) phyllodes tumour. A mammary tumour from a 62-year-old woman. There is an epithelial component, forming narrow, branching tubules. The surrounding stroma comprises closely packed, hyperchromatic, spheroidal and fusiform cells. Numerous mitotic figures could be seen at higher magnification within the stroma.   H & E × 96

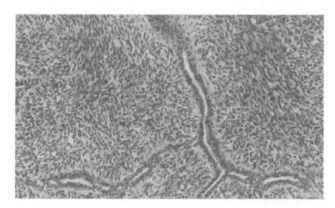

Figure 21.5 Malignant (cystosarcoma) phyllodes tumour. A tumour from the breast of a 49-year-old woman. The section shows both the epithelial component consisting of thin branching tubules, and the highly cellular malignant stroma featuring numerous mitotic figures.   H & E × 96

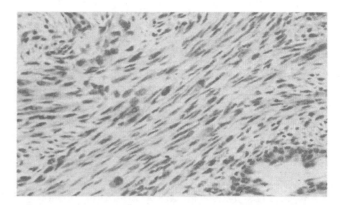

Figure 21.6 Malignant (cystosarcoma) phyllodes tumour. A tumour excised from the breast of a 59-year-old woman. Part of the epithelial component is present in the right lower corner of the photograph, but the field is dominated by a spindle cell sarcomatous stroma, featuring considerable nuclear pleomorphism.   H & E × 240

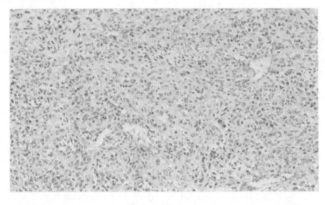

Figure 21.7 Mammary sarcoma; undifferentiated. A tumour excised from the breast of a 54-year-old woman. Much of the neoplasm had the typical microscopic structure of a phyllodes tumour, with regularly arranged epithelial and stromal components. In the area illustrated here, the stroma has outgrown the epithelium, and comprises an undifferentiated sarcoma. H & E × 96

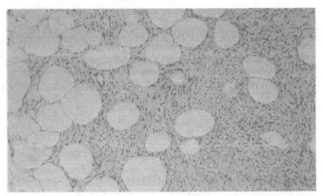

Figure 21.8 Malignant (cystosarcoma) phyllodes tumour: infiltrating edge. A section showing the periphery of a malignant phyllodes tumour with a fibro-sarcomatous pattern. The sarcoma has outgrown the epithelial component, and is infiltrating the fatty tissue of the breast. H & E × 96

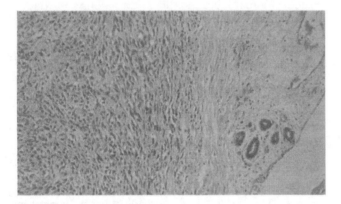

Figure 21.9 Malignant (cystosarcoma) phyllodes tumour: sharply defined periphery. In contrast to the invasive pattern illustrated in Figure 21.8, this tumour has a sharply defined edge, with a margin of compressed connective tissue between the cellular sarcoma on the left and the adjacent breast on the right of the photograph. H & E × 96

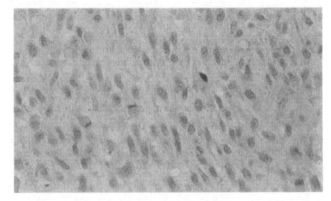

Figure 21.10 Malignant (cystosarcoma) phyllodes tumour. Section of a large tumour excised from the breast of a 60-year-old woman. The macroscopic appearances were those of a phyllodes tumour. Microscopically, much of the neoplasm appeared benign, but in one part the stroma was hyper-cellular and had outgrown the epithelial structures: this sarcomatous component is illustrated here. The histological pattern is that of a well-differ-entiated fibrosarcoma. Note the presence of mitotic figures. H & E × 240

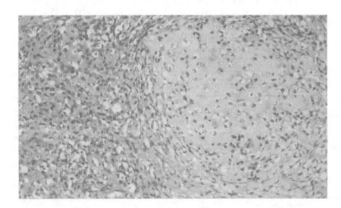

Figure 21.11 Mammary sarcoma with cartilage formation. Section of a recurrent breast tumour from a 48-year-old woman who had had a malignant phyllodes tumour excised 18 months before. The recurrent neoplasm lacked an epithelial component, and was entirely sarcomatous; it displayed fibro-sarcomatous growth, and also areas of osteoid, bone and cartilage formation. In this photograph, a mass of neoplastic cartilage occupies the right half of the field. H & E × 96

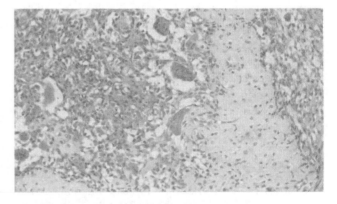

Figure 21.12 Mammary sarcoma with cartilage and giant cells. Another part of the tumour illustrated in Figure 21.11. In addition to islands of cartilage, there are multinucleated, osteoclast-like giant cells. H & E × 96

distinguish from an anaplastic carcinoma. The presence of metaplastic tissue in a malignant phyllodes tumour tends to indicate a more aggressive clinical course. Metaplasia may first appear in a recurrent neoplasm (Figures 21.11 and 21.12). The epithelial component of a phyllodes tumour, be it benign or malignant, may show marked hyperplasia (Figure 21.13). Squamous metaplasia can also occur (Figure 21.14). There are rare reports in the literature of carcinoma arising within the epithelial component[2,3,10].

Local recurrence occurs in about 20% of phyllodes tumours and is seen in both benign and malignant tumours[1-3]. It is probably due to inadequate local excision as very often these tumours have knob-like peripheral extensions, which may be left behind at the time of removal if the tumour is enucleated, and later give rise to recurrence. Detailed histological examination of all recurrent tumours is important, because a previously histologically benign neoplasm may recur as a malignant lesion[2]. A locally recurrent malignant tumour may have a benign epithelial component or be purely sarcomatous. Metastatic lesions consist only of the malignant stromal component. Metastasis via lymphatics is rare and spread usually occurs through the bloodstream. Therefore treatment should consist of simple mastectomy for malignant phyllodes tumours, and wide local excision (which may result in simple mastectomy in a small breast with a large tumour) for lesions considered to be benign. The commonest sites for secondary deposits from malignant phyllodes tumours are lung and bone, but metastases in the heart, intestinal tract, endocrine glands and subcutaneous tissue have all been recorded[1-4]. The reported incidence of metastases varies from 6 to 70% of phyllodes tumours[3], although the upper figure would appear to be too high. Metastasis probably occurs in approximately 25% of tumours which are malignant on histological examination[1]. Recurrence or metastasis usually develops within two years of the initial diagnosis; in cases where the tumour proves fatal, death generally occurs within five years[3,4]. However, there is considerable variation, and metastases have been reported as late as 12 years after diagnosis[2,3]. Malignant neoplasms can kill by direct extension into the chest wall without the development of metastases[1-4]. This is particularly likely to happen in patients receiving inadequate initial treatment, in whom local recurrence has taken place.

Pure Sarcoma of the Breast

Some mammary sarcomas have no associated epithelial component and thus no evidence that the tumour is part of a fibroepithelial neoplasm, although multiple block studies may be necessary to exclude the presence of an epithelial component. It must also be stressed that exhaustive sampling is essential to distinguish pure sarcomas from carcinomas exhibiting metaplasia (see Chapter 16).

Berg and colleagues[11] studied 86 primary sarcomas of the breast, the series comprising 40 malignant cysto-sarcoma phyllodes tumours, 14 malignant lymphomas, 7 angiosarcomas and 25 neoplasms which the authors designated stromal sarcomas. The stromal sarcomas were malignant connective-tissue tumours featuring fibroblasts and lipoblasts but no heterologous elements and no epithelial component. They stressed that microscopically the tumour tissue appeared to be analogous to the intralobular, interlobular and fatty components of the normal mammary connective tissue; implicit in their

description is the suggestion that they were observing an organ-specific sarcoma arising from the specialized stroma of the breast. Subsequent workers[12] have criticized the term stromal sarcoma on the assumption that it embraces all histological types of pure mammary sarcoma, excluding angiosarcoma and malignant lymphoma, and have advocated a classification of mammary sarcomas according to the same nomenclature as that used for malignant mesenchymal tumours in other anatomical sites. Whilst this proposition seems logical, as pointed out by Norris and Taylor[13], despite the general histological similarity of pure mammary sarcomas to malignant mesenchymal tumours elsewhere in the body, those in the breast are more prone to form bone, cartilage, muscle and fat. Although this is in contradistinction to the findings of Berg and colleagues[11] it does seem that pure sarcomas of the breast do have certain special features. Nevertheless, sub-division according to the main histological component is justified because it has prognostic significance: for example, tumours having a predominantly osteosarcomatous, chondrosarcomatous or rhabdomyosarcomatous pattern behave in a very aggressive fashion.

Pure mammary sarcomas are less common than malignant phyllodes tumours and occur in a slightly older age group: in one series the average age was 51 years[12]. They have a similar histological appearance to phyllodes tumours apart from the absence of the epithelial component. On gross examination the tumour usually consists of a grey or white, rubbery mass. Gritty foci, areas of cystic degeneration, haemorrhage and necrosis may be present. The average size varies from 3 to 6 cm[8,11-13]. The border may be well circumscribed or infiltrative. The commonest histological pattern is that of a fibrosarcoma (Figure 21.15), but, as already mentioned, metaplasia is common and may result in the formation of bone, cartilage, adipose tissue or rarely muscle (Figures 21.16 and 21.17). Furthermore, neoplasms having the pattern of a malignant fibrous histiocytoma, an anaplastic sarcoma or a malignant giant cell tumour of soft parts can occur (Figures 21.18–21.20). The presence of an infiltrative margin, severe cellular atypia and a high mitotic rate (5 or more per 10 high power fields) are strong indications that the tumour will recur or metastasize[12,13]. Treatment consists of simple mastectomy. Although, as with malignant phyllodes tumours, axillary lymph nodes are sometimes enlarged this is nearly always due to reactive changes and not metastases. Spread occurs via the blood stream, most frequently to lungs and bones. In a review of the literature Barnes and Pietruszka[12] found that 29% of patients died within 5 years of diagnosis.

Mammary sarcomas having a single uniform pattern throughout (e.g. pure liposarcoma, osteosarcoma or rhabdomyosarcoma) have been reported but extensive sampling is necessary to establish the purity of the lesion[7-9,14-16].

As is evident from the above discussion there is considerable confusion in the literature concerning the precise classification of pure mammary sarcomas and general agreement on terminology has not yet been established.

Postmastectomy Lymphangiosarcoma

In 1948 Stewart and Treves[17] reported a series of six patients in whom multinodular haemorrhagic tumours developed in arms affected by chronic lymphoedema.

The patients were all women who had undergone mastectomy which was followed by chronic lymphoedema of the upper limb on the same side. The interval between mastectomy and the appearance of the new tumours ranged from 6 to 24 years. Stewart and Treves considered the haemorrhagic neoplasms in the limbs to be lymphangiosarcomas, chronic oedema presumably being the main aetiological factor. Since its original description, the occurrence of this syndrome has become widely recognized, and many further cases have been reported. Furthermore, angiosarcomas have been found to arise in limbs affected by congenital and idiopathic lymphoedema, unassociated with pre-existing malignant disease[18]. Nevertheless, the angiosarcomatous nature of the neoplasms has been challenged, and it has been suggested that they represent multiple secondary carcinomas arising by retrograde spread in the oedematous limb[19]. Whilst it cannot be denied that this alternative histogenesis may apply in some cases, most workers consider the Stewart–Treves tumours to be vascular mesenchymal growths: some regard them as haemangiosarcomas, and some maintain that they are closely related to Kaposi's sarcoma. Additional support for an endothelial derivation of postmastectomy lymphangiosarcoma comes from ultrastructural and immunohistochemical studies. Miettinin and colleagues[20], in a study of two cases, demonstrated that the cells of the angiosarcomas gave positive reactions for endothelial markers, but reacted negatively with the epithelial marker. Furthermore when retrograde lymphatic spread from mammary carcinoma does occur, the epithelial nature of the metastasis is usually quite obvious microscopically (see Chapter 18, Figure 18.5).

Whatever its exact nature may be, the development of multiple haemorrhagic tumour masses in a chronically oedematous limb, often after many years of freedom from overt cancer, presents a characteristic and striking clinical syndrome (Figure 21.21). The prognosis is grave; in one review only 11 of 129 patients survived more than five years[18]. Widespread metastatic dissemination often occurs (Figure 21.22).

Radiation-induced Sarcoma

The carcinogenic effects of ionizing radiation have long been recognized. The radiation may be internal when radioactive substances are deposited in the tissues, or external as in conventional radiotherapy. The occurrence of sarcoma following radiotherapy for cancer of the breast is rare but well-documented. In a review of the literature, Young and Liebscher[21] found reports of 28 cases of bone sarcoma developing in mammary radiation fields, and recorded a further example. The bones involved include rib, scapula, clavicle, humerus and sternum. Most of the tumours were osteosarcomas, but some were classified as fibrosarcoma or chondrosarcoma, and a few were of unspecified type. The interval between radiotherapy and the appearance of the sarcoma ranged from 32 months to 42 years, with means of 10–16 years in different studies. The overall incidence of bone sarcoma after radiotherapy has been estimated to be 0.03%, with an even smaller incidence following irradiation for mammary carcinoma. An example is illustrated in Figures 21.23 and 21.24.

Sarcomas of soft tissue have also been reported to occur after radiotherapy for breast cancer. The recorded tumours include fibrosarcoma, malignant fibrous histiocytoma, liposarcoma and undifferentiated sarcoma[22].

Carcinosarcoma of the Breast

Composite tumours having malignant components of both epithelial and mesenchymal types (carcinosarcomas) are rare in the human breast. Some neoplasms which appear to be carcinosarcomas on initial examination prove to be carcinomas with metaplasia or a dedifferentiated spindle-cell (sarcomatoid) moiety when they are subjected to more critical and detailed study[2]. Nevertheless, true carcinosarcomas do occasionally occur. In a review of carcinosarcomas Harris and Persaud[23] found only 16 acceptable cases. The sarcomatous component can be fibroblastic, chondroid, osseous or even osteoclastic. As mentioned in Chapter 16 bone and cartilage may arise from carcinoma cells by metaplasia. Such tumours are not carcinosarcomas in the strict histogenetic sense of the term which should be reserved for mixed malignant neoplasms in which the non-epithelial components are of mesenchymal origin. The development of carcinoma from the epithelial component of both benign and malignant phyllodes tumours has already been mentioned.

References

1. Hart, W. R., Bauer, R. C. and Oberman, H. A. (1978). Cystosarcoma phyllodes: a clinicopathologic study of twenty-six hypercellular periductal stromal tumors of the breast. *Am. J. Clin. Pathol.*, **70**, 211–216

2. Azzopardi, J. G. (1979). *Problems in Breast Pathology*, p. 346. Vol. 11 in Bennington, J. L. (ed.) *Major Problems in Pathology*. (London, Philadelphia, Toronto: Saunders)

3. Rosenfeld, J. C., DeLaurentis, D. A. and Lerner, H. (1981). Cystosarcoma phyllodes. Diagnosis and management. *Cancer Clin. Trials*, **4**, 187–193

4. Pietruszka, M. and Barnes, L. (1978). Cystosarcoma phyllodes. A clinicopathologic analysis of 42 cases. *Cancer*, **41**, 1974–1983

5. Andersson, A. and Bergdahl, L. (1978). Cystosarcoma phyllodes in young women. *Arch. Surg.*, **113**, 742–744

6. Pantoja, E., Llobet, R. E. and Lopez, E. (1976). Gigantic cystosarcoma phyllodes in a man with gynecomastia. *Arch. Surg.*, **111**, 611

7. Rasmussen, J. and Jensen, H. (1979). Liposarcoma of the breast. Case report and review of the literature. *Virchows Arch. A Path. Anat. Histol.*, **385**, 117–124

8. Smith, B. H. and Taylor, H. B. (1969). The occurrence of bone and cartilage in mammary tumours. *Am. J. Clin. Pathol.*, **51**, 610–618

9. Barnes, L. and Pietruzka, M. (1978). Rhabdomyosarcoma arising within a cystosarcoma phyllodes. Case report and review of the literature. *Am. J. Surg. Pathol.*, **2**, 423–429

10. Klausner, J. M., Lelcuk, S., Ilia, B., Inbar, M., Hammer, B., Skornik, Y. and Rozin, R. R. (1983). Breast carcinoma originating in cystosarcoma phyllodes. *Clin. Oncol.*, **9**, 71–74

11. Berg, J. W., DeCrosse, J. J., Fracchia, A. A. and Farrow, J. (1962). Stromal sarcomas of the breast. *Cancer*, **15**, 418–424

12. Barnes, L. and Pietruszka, M. (1977). Sarcomas of the breast. A clinicopathologic analysis of ten cases. *Cancer*, **40**, 1577–1585

13. Norris, H. J. and Taylor, H. B. (1968). Sarcomas and related mesenchymal tumours of the breast. *Cancer*, **22**, 22–28

14. Inauen, W. and Gloor, F. J. (1981). Malignant giant cell tumour of the breast associated with infiltrating duct carcinoma. *Virchows Arch. (Pathol. Anat.)*, **393**, 359–364

15. Beltaos, E., Banerjee, T. K. (1979). Chondrosarcoma of the breast. Report of two cases. *Am. J. Clin. Pathol.*, **71**, 345–349

16. Chen, K. T. K., Kuo, T-T., Hoffmann, K. .D. (1981). Leiomyosarcoma of the breast. A case of long survival and late hepatic metastasis. *Cancer*, **47**, 1883–1886

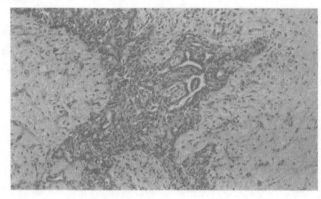

Figure 21.13 Malignant (cystosarcoma) phyllodes tumour with epithelial hyperplasia. The epithelium shows hyperplasia of both juxtaluminal and myoepithelial cells. The mesenchymal component although not very cellular in this field shows nuclear atypia and mitotic figures. Elsewhere in the tumour there was a definite sarcomatous pattern.   H & E × 96

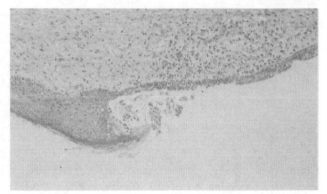

Figure 21.14 Squamous metaplasia in malignant (cystosarcoma) phyllodes tumour. On the left, the epithelium lining a cleft shows squamous metaplasia with keratinization. In this field, the mesenchymal component is not very cellular, but definite sarcomatous growth was present in other parts of the tumour.   H & E × 96

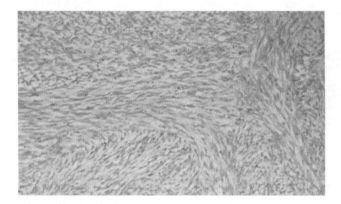

Figure 21.15 Fibrosarcoma of the breast. A large tumour from the breast of a 51-year-old woman. The growth was entirely sarcomatous, and the study of multiple tissue blocks failed to show any epithelial component. The neoplasm consists of interwoven fasciculi of fibroblasts, displaying a moderate number of mitotic figures.   H & E × 96

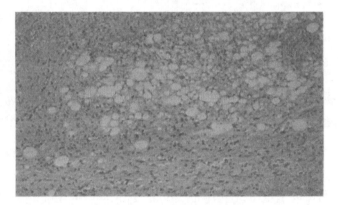

Figure 21.16 Mammary sarcoma with liposarcomatous areas. Section of a mammary tumour from a 46-year-old woman. Multiple block study failed to show an epithelial component. The neoplasm displays a blending of pleomorphic lipoblasts and small undifferentiated cells in a myxoid matrix. H & E × 96

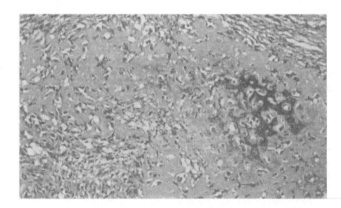

Figure 21.17 Mammary sarcoma with osteosarcomatous areas. Section of a mammary tumour from a 48-year-old woman. No epithelial component could be found, despite the study of multiple tissue blocks. The neoplasm is composed of pleomorphic spheroidal and fusiform cells and there is abundant tumour osteoid and bone.   H & E × 96

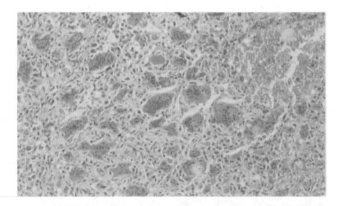

Figure 21.18 Mammary sarcoma with osteoclast-like giant cells. A sarcoma from the breast of a 66-year-old woman. No evidence of a phyllodes tumour could be found. In some areas there was tumour bone and cartilage formation. In the field shown here, there are numerous multinucleated giant cells similar to those seen in giant-cell tumours of bone. Pleomorphic, mononucleated sarcoma cells are present between the giant cells.   H & E × 96

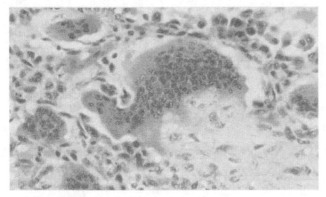

Figure 21.19 Mammary sarcoma with osteoclast-like giant cells. Higher magnification of the section illustrated in Figure 21.18, showing detail of the multinucleated giant cells and the interposed pleomorphic, mononuclear sarcoma cells. H & E × 240

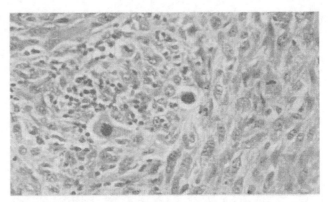

Figure 21.20 Mammary sarcoma with the pattern of a malignant fibrous histiocytoma. A tumour from the breast of a 47-year-old woman. No epithelial component could be demonstrated. The neoplasm consists of large, pleomorphic spheroidal and fusiform cells, displaying many mitotic figures and intermingled with lymphocytes and plasmacytes. In other areas there were large cells with foamy cytoplasm and bizarre nuclei, similar to those commonly seen in malignant fibrous histiocytoma in other anatomical sites. H & E × 240

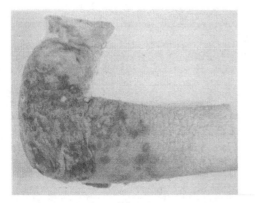

Figure 21.21 Lymphangiosarcoma in lymphoedematous arm. Part of an amputation specimen showing the multiple cutaneous nodules characteristic of the Stewart–Treves syndrome; some of the nodules have become confluent. The patient was a 61-year-old woman who had had a radical mastectomy and post-operative radiotherapy for breast carcinoma 11 years previously. Since the time of treatment her arm had been swollen with lymphoedema. She noticed the red cutaneous nodules about 4 months before amputation. She died with disseminated malignant disease 18 months later

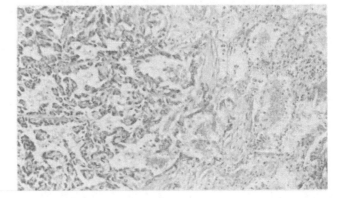

Figure 21.22 Secondary lymphangiosarcoma of the lung in Stewart–Treves syndrome. The secondary angiosarcoma occupies the left half of the field; it forms vascular spaces and irregular tufts of endothelial cells. The patient was a 69-year-old woman who had had a lymphoedematous arm for 9 years following radical treatment for mammary carcinoma. She developed clinical features of postmastectomy lymphangiosarcoma similar to those illustrated in Figure 21.21. She died with disseminated angiosarcoma one year later. H & E × 96

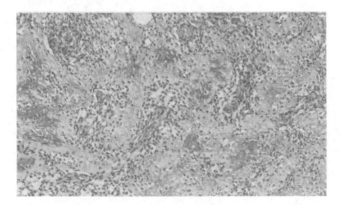

Figure 21.23 Radiation-induced osteosarcoma of sternum. Section of a sternal neoplasm arising in a 60-year-old woman 12 years after post-operative radiotherapy for mammary carcinoma. The sternum was excised, but the patient died from recurrent osteosarcoma 2 years later. The photomicrograph shows darkly-staining spheroidal and fusiform sarcoma cells within a plexus of abundant tumour osteoid and bone. H & E × 96

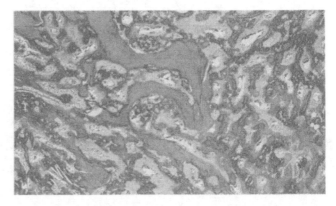

Figure 21.24 Radiation-induced osteosarcoma of sternum. Another part of the tumour illustrated in Figure 21.23. Here, sarcoma cells are relatively sparse, but tumour osteoid and bone are abundant, and have replaced the marrow between the normal cancellous trabeculae. H & E × 96

17. Stewart, F. W. and Treves, N. (1948). Lymphangiosarcoma in postmastectomy lymphedema: a report of six cases in elephantiasis chirurgica. *Cancer,* **1**, 64–81

18. Woodward, A. H., Ivins, J. C. and Soule, E. H. (1972). Lymphangiosarcoma arising in chronic lymphedematous extremities. *Cancer,* **30**, 562–572

19. Schafler, K., McKenzie, C. G. and Salm, R. (1979). Postmastectomy lymphangiosarcoma: a reappraisal of the concept – a critical review and report of an illustrative case. *Histopathology,* **3**, 131–152

20. Miettinen, M., Lehto, V-P. and Virtanen, I. (1983). Postmastectomy angiosarcoma (Stewart–Treves syndrome). Light-microscopic, immunohistological, and ultrastructural characteristics of two cases. *Am. J. Surg. Pathol.,* **7**, 329–339

21. Young, J. W. and Liebscher, L. A. (1982). Postirradiation osteogenic sarcoma with unilateral metastatic spread within the field of irradiation. *Skeletal Radiol.,* **8**, 279–283

22. Arbabi, L. and Warhol, M. J. (1982). Pleomorphic liposarcoma following radiotherapy for breast carcinoma. *Cancer,* **49**, 878–880

23. Harris, M. and Persaud, V. (1974). Carcinosarcoma of the breast. *J. Pathol.,* **112**, 99–105

Angiosarcoma

22

The term angiosarcoma encompasses both haemangio-sarcoma and lymphangiosarcoma but, in respect of mammary neoplasms, the short term angiosarcoma has been used as a synonym for haemangiosarcoma.

Mammary angiosarcoma has generally been considered to be a highly lethal neoplasm, only 14% of patients remaining disease free for 3 years in a collected series up to 1980[1]. However, more recent reports have recorded higher survival rates, and have described different histological patterns of angiosarcoma which can be correlated with prognosis[2,3].

Angiosarcoma usually presents as a painless mass which may grow rapidly. Bluish discoloration is noted in the overlying skin of some patients. On gross examination, the tumour consists of poorly defined spongy haemorrhagic tissue. There may be areas of thickening and induration and microscopic sections usually show extension of the neoplasm well beyond the apparent gross margins of the tumour. Although often diagnosed clinically as carcinoma, almost half the cases recorded in the literature have been initially diagnosed histologically as benign lesions, such as angioma, organizing thrombus, organizing haematoma or granulation tissue. The very rarity of angiosarcoma of the breast has tended to perpetuate this error through ignorance of the deceptively benign microscopic pattern which it often presents. Any mammary tissue with an angiomatous component should be viewed with suspicion, and widely sampled for histological examination, since unequivocally malignant areas may be extremely small. Microscopically, angiosarcomas are composed of anastomosing vascular channels which are often thin-walled and lined by well-differentiated endothelial cells (Figure 22.1). However, a thorough search of the neoplasm should reveal small foci in which the endothelial cells display malignant characteristics, such as hyperchromasia and increased mitotic activity (Figure 22.2). Tumours which display only these characteristics have been found by Donnell and colleagues[2] to be associated with a good prognosis and have been designated Group 1. In their study, 10 of 13 patients in this histological group were alive and free from disease after an average follow-up of nearly 6 years. Well-formed vascular channels are seen around the periphery of most angiosarcomas but towards the centre there may be areas of marked endothelial proliferation resulting in tufting and papillary projections into the lumina of the vascular spaces (Figures 22.3, 22.4, 22.7 and 22.9). Occasionally the capillaries may be reduced to slits within an almost solid growth of malignant endothelial cells showing large numbers of mitoses (Figures 22.5, 22.6, 22.8 and 22.10). Where this pattern predominated, especially in the presence of blood lakes and necrosis, Donnell et al.[2] designated the tumours Group 3 and found them to be associated with

logical pattern. Donnell et al.[2] also found that the size of the tumour was of significance and that disease-free patients had an average tumour size of 4 cm, compared a poor prognosis. Only 2 of 18 patients in this histological group were free of disease 11 and 5 years respectively after diagnosis and treatment. A small intermediate group with a histological pattern between the two extremes was designated Group 2, and patients with tumours in this group had a survival rate similar to those with the more favourable Group 1 histological pattern. Donnell et al.[2] also found that the size of the tumour was of significance and that disease-free patients had an average tumour size of 4 cm, compared with 6.5 cm in those who died of their disease.

In a similar subsequent study, Merino et al.[3] divided angiosarcomas into well-differentiated, moderately differentiated and poorly differentiated tumours. They also found a close correlation between histological type and prognosis. Four of their five patients with well-differentiated lesions remained free from disease for as long as 24 years. Three of four patients with moderately differentiated lesions and three of six with poorly differentiated tumours died of the disease at intervals up to 4 years.

The diagnosis of angiosarcoma should present no difficulty in the presence of obviously malignant endothelium, particularly with a solid growth pattern, but such areas may be inconspicuous and it is wise policy to regard all angiomatous lesions of the breast as probably malignant unless they fulfil the strict criteria for a benign angioma. Although benign angiomas do occur they are extremely rare and usually very small.

Local recurrence is common with angiosarcoma. Metastases occur via the blood stream rather than lymphatics and are most frequently seen in lungs, bone, liver, skin and brain. Treatment should consist of thorough surgical excision of the tumour which will necessitate simple mastectomy in most cases. Axillary metastases are rare, so axillary dissection would appear to be unnecessary. In their study Donnell et al.[2] reported improved prognosis with the use of adjuvant actino-mycin D.

Ultrastructural and histochemical studies of angiosarcomas have confirmed the endothelial nature of the neoplastic cells, but also indicate a transition to pericytes and undifferentiated mesenchymal cells in some areas; these features have also been described in angiosarcomas in other organs[4]. Merino et al.[3] found that immunoperoxidase staining for factor VIII related antigen was markedly positive in cells lining the vascular channels of well-differentiated tumours; it was present but less intensely positive in poorly differentiated areas of angiosarcomas.

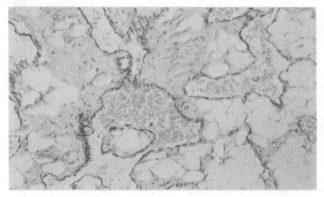

Figure 22.1 Angiosarcoma of the breast. A tumour from the breast of a 23-year-old woman. In this field the neoplasm comprises thin-walled, dilated, anastomosing vascular channels, ramifying amongst fibro-fatty tissue. Such a well-differentiated growth pattern may lead to a false diagnosis of benignity: multiple block study is mandatory for all angiomatous lesions of the breast. H & E × 96

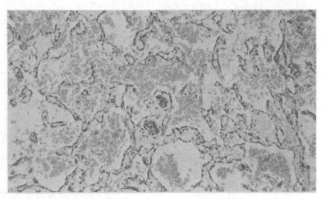

Figure 22.2 Angiosarcoma of the breast. A tumour from the breast of a 22-year-old woman. Two small mammary ducts are present near the centre of the field. The neoplasm forms wide, anastomosing vascular channels. The endothelial cells are disposed mainly as single layers, but some are large and hyperchromatic. H & E × 96

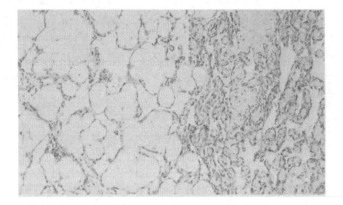

Figure 22.3 Angiosarcoma of the breast. A tumour from the breast of a 37-year-old woman. This field shows the juxtaposition of two patterns: anastomosing thin-walled vascular channels on the left, and papillary formations on the right. H & E × 96

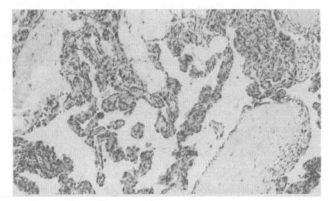

Figure 22.4 Angiosarcoma of the breast. Another part of the tumour illustrated in Figure 22.1. The proliferating neoplastic endothelium forms complex papillary tufts projecting into the lumina of the vascular spaces. H & E × 96

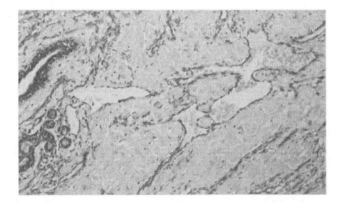

Figure 22.5 Angiosarcoma of the breast. A further section of the tumour illustrated in Figures 22.1 and 22.4. Here, the sarcoma has formed irregularly-shaped, wide, anastomosing vascular channels in the fibrous tissues of the breast. A duct and part of a lobule are present on the extreme left. H & E × 96

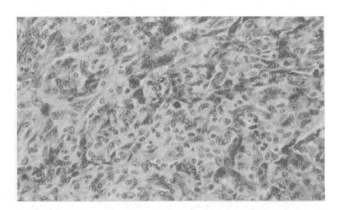

Figure 22.6 Angiosarcoma of the breast. Another part of the tumour illustrated in Figures 22.1, 22.4 and 22.5. Here, the neoplasm is highly cellular, displays mitotic activity and is poorly vasoformative. H & E × 240

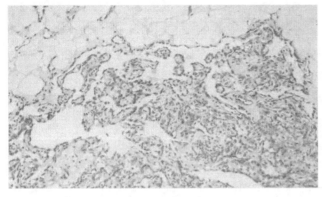

Figure 22.7 Angiosarcoma of the breast. Section showing a large vascular channel with complex papillary ingrowths of neoplastic endothelium. H & E × 96

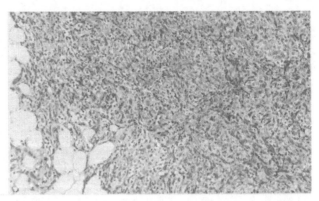

Figure 22.8 Angiosarcoma of the breast. Another section of the tumour illustrated in Figure 22.7. In this area, the sarcoma cells are closely packed into solid masses, although a few inconspicuous slit-like vascular spaces can be seen here and there. H & E × 96

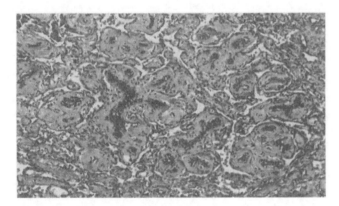

Figure 22.9 Angiosarcoma of the breast. Sections showing a mammary lobule expanded and disorganized by a labyrinth of vascular channels. The vessels are lined by hyperchromatic, malignant endothelial cells. H & E × 96

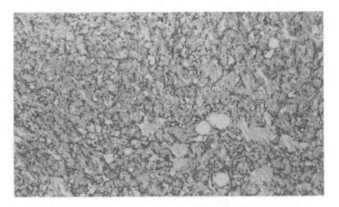

Figure 22.10 Angiosarcoma of the breast. This tumour displays a complex mesh of intercommunicating, thin-walled vascular channels, lined by prominent neoplastic endothelial cells and with erythrocytes in the lumina. H & E × 96

References

1. Chen, K. T. K., Kirkegaard, D. D. and Bocian, J. J. (1980). Angiosarcoma of the breast. *Cancer*, **46**, 368–371

2. Donnell, R. M., Rosen, P. P., Lieberman, P. H., Kaufman, R. J., Kay, S., Braun, D. W. Jr. and Kinne, D. W. (1981). Angiosarcoma and other vascular tumors of the breast. Pathologic analysis as a guide to prognosis. *Am. J. Surg. Pathol.*, **5**, 629–642

3. Merino, M. J., Carter, D. and Berman, M. (1983). Angiosarcoma of the breast. *Am. J. Surg. Pathol.*, **7**, 53–60

4. Alvarez-Fernandez, E. and Salinero-Paniagua, E. (1981). Vascular tumours of the mammary gland. A histochemical and ultrastructural study. *Virchows Arch. (Pathol. Anat.)*, **394**, 31–47

23

Lymphoma and Leukaemia

Lymphoma of the Breast

The breast is not uncommonly involved in patients with disseminated lymphoma or leukaemia; rarely lymphoma appears to arise primarily within the breast. Secondary involvement can occur with any type of lymphoma, including Hodgkin's disease. The tumour deposits present as either single or multiple nodules and are frequently bilateral. On gross and mammographic examination, the neoplasm usually appears well-circumscribed although diffuse involvement can occur[1]. Microscopically the outline is generally less sharp and tumour cells may be seen streaming out into the surrounding tissue. The overall appearances are similar to those of lymphomatous deposits at other sites. The glandular tissue of the breast is frequently preserved, although surrounded and compressed by the lymphomatous infiltrate. Treatment and prognosis depend on the type and extent of the disease.

Primary lymphoma of the breast (that is lymphoma apparently confined to the breast or to the breast and regional lymph nodes) is much less common and accounts for only about 0.1% of all malignant mammary tumours, if strict criteria are applied to its diagnosis. Various different histological types of malignant lymphoma arising primarily in the breast have been reported, the majority being of non-Hodgkin's type. In most series the tumours have been specified according to the Rappaport, or a modified Rappaport, classification. They include lymphomas of diffuse histiocytic, nodular or diffuse well-differentiated lymphocytic, nodular or diffuse poorly-differentiated lymphocytic, lymphoblastic and undifferentiated types[2-4]. As with secondary lymphoma, the patient usually presents with a rapidly growing mass. Skin fixation, oedema of the breast, *peau d'orange*, increased warmth and redness of the skin have all been described[1-4]. The lesion may be either unilateral or bilateral and in some series a predilection for involvement of the right breast has been found[2,3]. The age range is the same as for patients with carcinoma and clinically the lesion is almost invariably diagnosed as carcinoma. The histological appearances are similar in both primary and secondary lymphoma (Figures 23.1–23.3). The prognosis of primary lymphoma of the breast as reported in the literature is variable and depends to some extent on the histological type of the lymphoma. However, it is generally considered to be poor, with eventual dissemination of disease in most patients. In the past, patients were generally treated by mastectomy with or without radiotherapy and chemotherapy. In more recent studies, however, treatment has consisted of a combination of radiotherapy and chemotherapy, usually without mastectomy[2-4].

Extra-medullary Plasmacytoma

Extra-medullary plasmacytoma also occurs in the breast[5,6] and may on rare occasions prove to be the first manifestation of an already disseminated disease (myelomatosis), as in the lesion illustrated in Figures 23.4–23.6.

Leukaemic Involvement of the Breast

Breast involvement can occur during the course of any type of leukaemia, including lymphocytic, lymphoblastic and myeloid varieties[1,7-9]. In some patients mammary involvement antedates or coincides with the diagnosis of the disease. The lesion may present as a diffuse involvement or as a localized mass[1]. In myeloid leukaemia the mass may have the characteristic green colour of a classic chloroma[7]. On histological examination as shown in Figures 23.7–23.10, the infiltrating leukaemic cells usually surround preserved ducts and lobules.

The diagnosis of lymphomatous or leukaemic involvement of the breast should present no problem in a patient with disseminated disease. However, in the case of a primary lymphoma, or a leukaemic deposit antedating overt generalized disease, differentiation from mammary carcinoma may be difficult. The pathologist should always bear in mind the possibility that a malignant neoplasm in the breast may be other than a primary carcinoma. Ultrastructural studies and special stains may be helpful. The demonstration of mucin in the malignant cells is indicative of a carcinoma. Immunoperoxidase staining for immunoglobulins may help in the diagnosis of lymphoma by demonstrating the monoclonal nature of the cells. The chloroacetate esterase technique is of value in identifying myeloid cells such as those in a deposit of granulocytic leukaemia (Figure 23.11). However, it should be noted that myeloid metaplasia can present as a breast mass in patients with myelofibrosis[10]. This should not be mistaken for malignant lymphoreticular disease or other neoplasms.

It is of interest that an association between acute leukaemia and mammary carcinoma has been noted. In one study a sevenfold increased incidence of acute leukaemia was found in patients with breast cancer[11]. It is not known whether this is related to the known increased risk of a second neoplasm developing in patients already having one primary tumour or if the leukaemia is related to radiotherapy or chemotherapy used in the treatment of breast carcinoma[11,12].

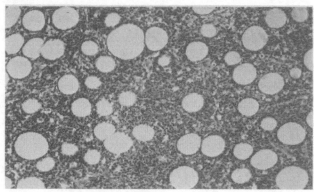

Figure 23.1 Malignant lymphoma of the breast. A mass from the breast of a 45-year-old woman. Investigations failed to reveal evidence of any disease elsewhere. The lymphoma cells show the characteristic diffuse pattern of infiltration in the mammary adipose tissue. H & E × 96

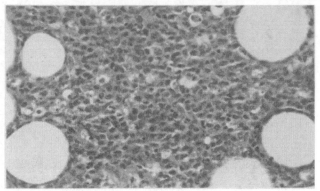

Figure 23.2 Malignant lymphoma of the breast. Higher magnification of the tumour illustrated in Figure 23.1. The neoplasm was classified as a non-Hodgkin's lymphoma, undifferentiated type. H & E × 240

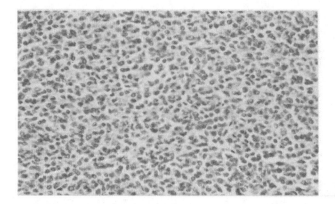

Figure 23.3 Malignant lymphoma of the breast. A mass from the breast of a 51-year-old woman. At the time of presentation, no involvement of other sites could be demonstrated, but a year later a similar tumour appeared in the opposite breast. The cells are loosely arranged and the nuclei are pleomorphic. The neoplasm was classified as a diffuse, follicular-centre cell (centroblastic) lymphoma. H & E × 240

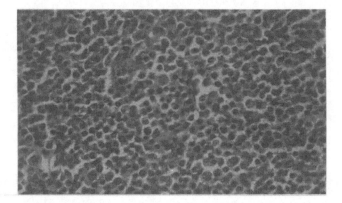

Figure 23.4 Plasmacytoma of the breast. The patient was a 63-year-old woman who presented with a mass in the left breast. Radiological examination showed an osteolytic lesion in the scapula, and the clinical diagnosis was mammary carcinoma with skeletal deposits. Later, an elevated monoclonal IgG was demonstrated in the plasma. The tumour is composed of moderately differentiated neoplastic plasmacytes, some of which display eccentric nuclei with peripheral chromatin stippling ('clock-face' appearance). H & E × 240

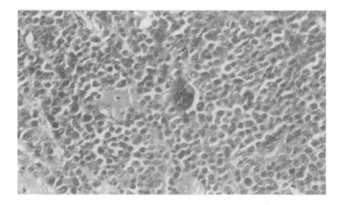

Figure 23.5 Plasmacytoma of the breast. A further section of the neoplasm illustrated in Figure 23.4, showing a tumour giant-cell at the centre of the field. H & E × 240

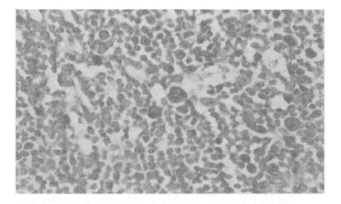

Figure 23.6 Plasmacytoma of the breast. A further section of the lesion illustrated in Figures 23.4 and 23.5, demonstrating cytoplasmic pyroninophilia. At the centre of the field there is a multinucleated tumour cell with prominent nucleoli. Methyl green/pyronin × 240

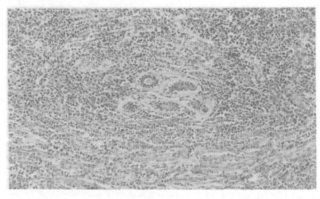

Figure 23.7 Myeloblastoma (granulocytic sarcoma) of the breast. Section of a mass from the breast of a 17-year-old girl. Macroscopically, the tumour was greenish: a classical chloroma. Acute myeloblastic leukaemia supervened within a few weeks. A small cluster of mammary ducts is present at the centre of the field, and the surrounding tissues are diffusely infiltrated with loosely-arranged, primitive myeloblasts. A few of the cells reacted positively to the chloroacetate esterase technique.   H & E × 96

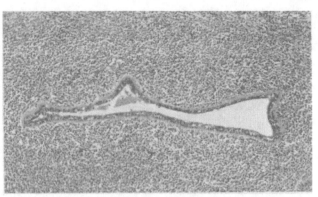

Figure 23.8 Myeloblastoma (granulocytic sarcoma) of the breast. A mass from the breast of a 22-year-old woman. Three months after excision of the mass, the patient developed the clinical and haematological features of acute myeloblastic leukaemia. The section shows a mammary duct surrounded by diffusely-arranged spheroidal cells.   H & E × 96

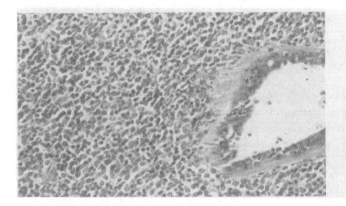

Figure 23.9 Myeloblastoma (granulocytic sarcoma) of the breast. Higher magnification of the lesion illustrated in Figure 23.8. The periductal tissues are infiltrated by primitive leukaemic myeloblasts.   H & E × 240

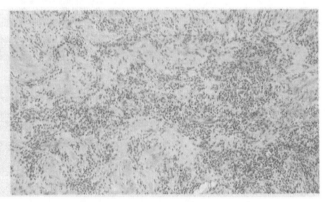

Figure 23.10 Myeloblastoma (granulocytic sarcoma) of the breast. Another section of the tumour shown in Figures 23.8 and 23.9. Here the leukaemic cells are infiltrating fibrous mammary stroma.   H & E × 96

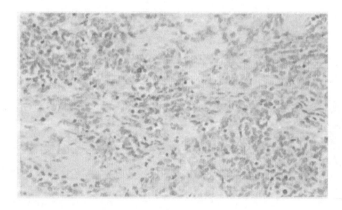

Figure 23.11 Myeloblastoma (granulocytic sarcoma) of the breast. A further section from the tumour illustrated in Figures 23.8–23.10, stained by chloroacetate esterase technique. Most of the cells are too primitive to react, but a few, such as the one near the centre of the field, have given a positive reaction and their cytoplasm is coloured red. Naphthol-AS-D-Chloroacetate esterase technique × 240

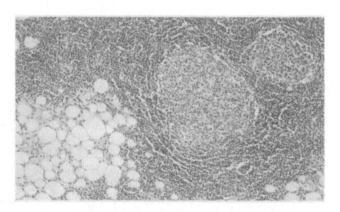

Figure 23.12 Pseudolymphoma of the breast. A lump excised from the breast of a 60-year-old woman. The lesion comprises an unencapsulated mass of lymphoid tissue, displaying prominent reaction centres. The absence of a capsule and sinusoids distinguishes a pseudolymphoma from an intra-mammary lymph node.   H & E × 96

Pseudolymphoma of the Breast

The differential diagnosis of a lymphoreticular disease of the breast also includes pseudolymphoma, although this lesion is rarely manifest in the breast. As in other sites, pseudolymphoma is characterized by a polymorphic cellular pattern and the presence of reaction centres (Figure 23.12). In addition the diagnosis can be supported by marker studies to demonstrate a mixed population of T and B lymphocytes, and the presence of cells with kappa and lambda light chains, in contrast to the monoclonal cytological population characteristic of a malignant lymphoma[13]. In a recent study, Lin and colleagues[14] reported on five cases of pseudolymphoma which accounted for 0.08% of all benign breast lesions they reviewed and 0.06% of all breast masses studied. The patients ranged from 26 to 57 years old with a mean age of 36 years. Clinically the tumours presented as a breast mass with a dull aching sensation in four patients. The duration of symptoms ranged from 2 weeks to 2 years. A history of physical trauma was present in three patients. After local excision none of the patients had a recurrence over a period of 2–8 years.

References

1. Millis, R. R., Atkinson, M. K. and Tonge, K. A. (1976). The xeroradiographic appearances of some uncommon malignant mammary neoplasms. Clin. Radiol., 27, 463–471
2. Mambo, N. C., Burke, J. S. and Butler, J. J. (1977). Primary malignant lymphomas of the breast. Cancer, 39, 2033–2040
3. Schouten, J. T., Weese, J. L. and Carbone, P. P. (1981). Lymphoma of the breast. Ann. Surg., 194, 749–753
4. Carbone, A., Volpe, R., Tirelli, U., Veronesi, A., Galligioni, E., Trovo, M. G. and Grigoletto, E. (1982). Primary lyphoblastic lymphoma of the breast. Clin. Oncol., 8, 367–373
5. Proctor, N. S. F., Rippey, J. J., Shulman, G. and Cohen, C. (1975). Extramedullary plasmacytoma of the breast. J. Pathol., 116, 97–100
6. Bassett, W. B. and Weiss, R. B. (1979). Plasmacytomas of the breast: An unusual manifestation of multiple myeloma. South. Med. J., 72, 1492–1494
7. Gralnick, H. R. and Dittmar, K. (1969). Development of myeloblastoma with massive breast and ovarian involvement during remission in acute leukaemia. Cancer, 24, 746–749
8. Kennedy, J., Bornstein, R., Brunning, R D. and Oines, D. (1970). Breast involvement in acute lymphatic leukemia. Cancer, 25, 693–696
9. O'Donnell, J. R. and Farrell, M. A. (1980). Acute myelogenous leukaemia with bilateral mammary gland involvement. J. Clin. Pathol., 33, 547–550
10. Brooks, J. J., Krugman, D. T. and Damjanov, I. (1980). Myeloid metaplasia presenting as a breast mass. Am. J. Surg. Pathol., 4, 281–285
11. Rosner, F., Carey, R. W. and Zarrabi, M. H. (1978). Breast cancer and acute leukemia. Report of 24 cases and review of literature. Am. J. Hematol., 4, 151–172
12. Ershler, W. B., Robins, H. I., Davis, H. L., Hafez, G.-R., Meisner, L. F., Dahlberg, S. and Arndt, C. (1982). Emergence of acute non-lymphocytic leukaemia in breast cancer patients. Am. J. Med. Sci., 284, 23–31
13. Fisher, E. R., Palekar, A. S., Paulson, J. D. and Golinger, R. (1979). Pseudolymphoma of the breast. Cancer, 44, 258–263
14. Lin, J. J., Farha, G. J. and Taylor, R. J. (1980). Pseudolymphoma of the breast. Cancer, 45, 973–978

Secondary tumours in the breast account for only a small proportion of all malignant mammary neoplasms but they are nevertheless important because they are often misdiagnosed. The most common secondary tumour is a metastasis from carcinoma of the contralateral breast, but this has to be distinguished from a new primary tumour. A metastasis from the contralateral breast may produce widespread lymphatic permeation, often initially involving the subdermal lymphatics, with multiple foci of invasion; such a lesion presents no problem. However, when there is a single nodule of invasive tumour the distinction can be extremely difficult and a definite diagnosis of a second primary tumour should only be made if (1) the second tumour is of a different type from the first, (2) the second tumour if of the same type is better differentiated than the first or (3) the second tumour has foci of in situ carcinoma contiguous with the infiltrating tumour. However, it should be recognized that in situ carcinoma can be present in addition to a metastatic infiltrating tumour from the opposite breast.

Metastatic involvement by other solid tumours excluding lymphoma and leukaemia accounts for about 0.25% of all malignant mammary neoplasms diagnosed in life although the incidence is higher in autopsy series[2]. The male breast may also be involved by metastatic solid tumours, but far less frequently than the female. It must also be emphasized that dual primaries consisting of a breast carcinoma and a primary tumour in another organ are distinctly more common than a primary tumour elsewhere metastasizing to the breast[1]. The primary tumours which most often metastasize to the breast are oat cell carcinoma of the bronchus and malignant melanoma (Figures 24.1 and 24.2). In a review of the literature on secondary tumours in the breast McIntosh and colleagues[1] found that bronchial carcinoma and malignant melanoma accounted for almost 50% of reported cases. However, metastases from many other tumours have been reported, including carcinoma of the prostate, gastrointestinal tract (including carcinoid tumours as illustrated in Figure 24.3), ovary, cervix uteri, endometrium, kidney, thyroid and urinary bladder and also such rarities as leiomyosarcoma (Figure 24.4), choriocarcinoma of the ovary (Figures 24.5 and 24.6), thymoma, angioblastic meningioma and cerebral astrocytoma[1-6]. Indeed almost any type of tumour can give rise to metastases in the breast.

Metastatic tumours may be single or multiple and usually consist of rounded or multinodular masses which are freely mobile within the breast. They are often mistaken for benign tumours on mammography (Figure 24.7), but rapid growth, which is frequently observed, should arouse suspicion of malignancy[1,4]. Microscopic recognition that the tumour is metastatic should present

no problem when the lesion is obviously foreign to the breast, for example a metastatic oat cell carcinoma, or when it displays a specific feature such as melanin pigment in a secondary malignant melanoma. This should not be confused with colonization by melanocytes of primary breast carcinomas involving the skin as illustrated in Figures 24.8 and 24.9[7]. However, an anaplastic secondary tumour can easily be misdiagnosed as a poorly differentiated primary mammary carcinoma. Metastatic tumours are usually well demarcated from the surrounding breast tissue on both gross and histological examination (Figure 24.10). Less commonly the growth pattern is more diffuse with periductal and perilobular spread (but without epithelial atypia in the ducts and lobules). Occasionally there is lymphatic permeation[3]. The absence of in situ carcinoma is another feature which should suggest the possibility of a secondary rather than a primary tumour. Stroma is not usually prominent, and elastosis has not been reported within metastatic tumours. Calcification is unusual but has been found in a few cases of metastatic ovarian carcinoma[4]. Finally, the histological similarity of a secondary deposit to a previously diagnosed primary tumour elsewhere will confirm the diagnosis. However, occasionally a metastatic tumour in the breast is the first manifestation of a primary neoplasm at another site. In seven of 29 cases described by McIntosh et al.[1], the breast lesion was the presenting feature of an occult neoplasm elsewhere, and in a further nine it was the first and only metastasis from a known primary. Immunohistochemical stains and electron microscopy may prove helpful in differentiating between primary and secondary carcinoma of the breast and, in the case of a secondary tumour, in identifying the primary site. For example, Choudhury et al.[8] identified a carcinoma of the male breast as primary, rather than metastatic from the prostate, by demonstrating the absence of prostatic acid phosphatase and prostatic antigen by immunohistochemical techniques. This is particularly pertinent in patients with prostatic carcinoma treated with oestrogens in whom it has been suggested that there is an increased risk of primary mammary carcinoma, and in whom secondary deposits of the prostatic tumour not infrequently develop in the breast[9]. Finally, the presence of oestrogen and progesterone receptors in a tumour would be supporting evidence for its origin within the breast although it should be remembered that other tumours can also contain hormone receptors.

Metastases from Primary Mammary Carcinomas

On rare occasions a mammary carcinoma first presents as a metastasis outside the breast, and pathologists

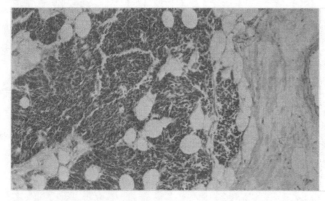

Figure 24.1 Oat cell carcinoma of bronchus, metastatic to breast. Section of a breast lump excised from a woman in whom a radiological diagnosis of bronchial carcinoma had been made. Although not encapsulated, the tumour deposit has a sharply defined edge. The cytological features are typical of an oat cell carcinoma.   H & E × 96

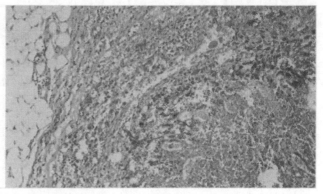

Figure 24.2 Malignant melanoma, metastatic to breast. Section of a breast lump from a woman who had had a cutaneous melanoma excised 2 years before. Although not encapsulated, the tumour deposit is quite sharply demarcated from the mammary adipose tissue on the left. There is extensive necrosis. A considerable amount of melanin pigment is present.   H & E × 96

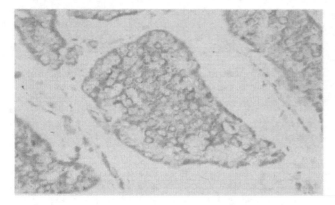

Figure 24.3 Ileal primary carcinoid, metastatic to breast. A breast lump from a woman who was known to have an ileal carcinoid with secondary deposits in the liver. The section shows the typical 'insular' pattern of a midgut carcinoid, with numerous argentaffin granules. Grimelius silver technique × 96

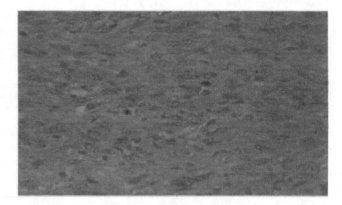

Figure 24.4 Leiomyosarcoma, metastatic to breast. Section of a mass from the breast of a woman who had had a hysterectomy for a uterine leiomyosarcoma 3 years before. The tumour deposit shown here is a moderately differentiated leiomyosarcoma. Note the mitotic figures.   H & E × 240

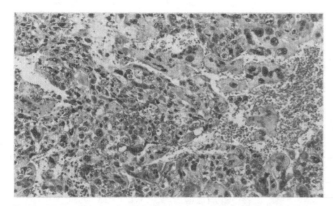

Figure 24.5 Choriocarcinoma, metastatic to breast. The patient was a 63-year-old woman who presented with a lump in the breast. Subsequently, she was found to have an ovarian teratoma with a choriocarcinomatous component. This is a section of the breast lesion. It shows the typical combination of cytotrophoblast and syncytiotrophoblast, with haemorrhage.   H & E × 240

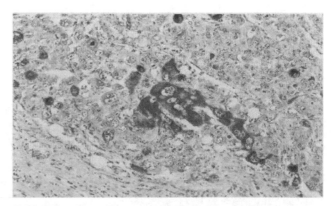

Figure 24.6 Choriocarcinoma, metastatic to breast. A further section of the tumour illustrated in Figure 24.5, stained by the immunoperoxidase technique for HCG. As indicated by the brown stain, HCG is located mainly in the syncytiotrophoblast. Immunoperoxidase technique for HCG × 240

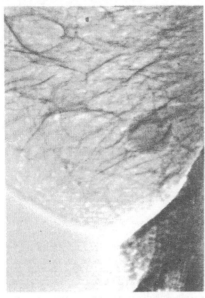

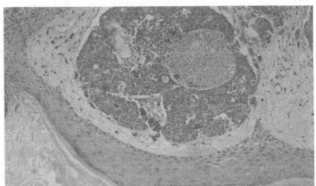

Figure 24.7 Oat cell carcinoma, metastatic to breast. A xeromammogram of the breast of a 63-year-old woman showing a well demarcated, rounded lesion in the breast resembling a fibroadenoma. This patient, however, had had an oat cell carcinoma of the bronchus diagnosed 6 months previously and the mammary lesion proved to be a secondary deposit

Figure 24.8 Melanin pigmentation of mammary carcinoma invading skin. Poorly differentiated duct carcinoma of the breast has infiltrated the dermis forming a large mass of cohesive carcinoma cells. The tumour cells are pleomorphic and display a number of mitotic figures; some contain brown granules. The pigment gives the staining reactions of melanin. H & E × 96

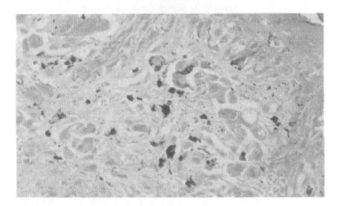

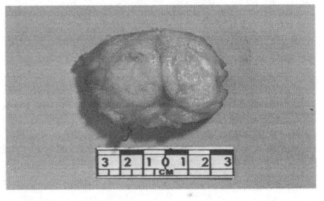

Figure 24.9 Melanin pigmentation of mammary carcinoma invading skin. A further section of the tumour illustrated in Figure 24.8. In this silver preparation, blackened melanin granules can be seen in some carcinoma cells and dendritic melanocytes are also demonstrated. Masson-Fontana × 240

Figure 24.10 Bronchial carcinoma, metastatic to breast. Bisected mass excised from the breast of a woman who was known to have an oat cell carcinoma of lung. The tumour deposit is spheroidal, well circumscribed, pinkish-grey and soft.

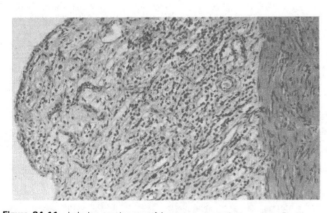

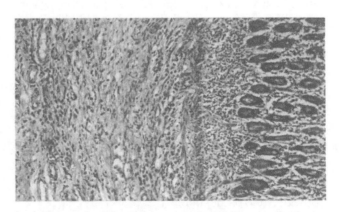

Figure 24.11 Lobular carcinoma of breast, metastatic to colon. Section showing marked thickening of the serosa; part of the colonic muscle is present on the right. The serosa is infiltrated with loosely-arranged small, hyperchromatic cells; some are lymphocytes but larger carcinoma cells are scattered amongst them. The patient presented with abdominal symptoms, part of the colon was resected and an initial diagnosis of malignant lymphoma was made. H & E × 96

Figure 24.12 Lobular carcinoma of breast, metastatic to colon. Another part of the colonic lesion illustrated in Figure 24.11. The mucosa is on the right. The submucosa is broadened and is infiltrated by widely scattered carcinoma cells. These cells are rather inconspicuous; they are best demonstrated by mucin stains. H & E × 96

should always be alert to this possibility. Even in patients with known mammary primaries this information is not always given by the clinician. Metastatic tumour in the gastrointestinal tract is not uncommon particularly from a primary lobular carcinoma, and can produce a variety of symptoms often simulating other diseases[10-12]. The lesion illustrated in Figures 24.11–24.13 shows metastatic lobular carcinoma of the breast in a colon. This patient underwent a hemicolectomy in the belief that she had a primary colonic tumour. A lump in the breast which proved on biopsy to be carcinoma was only found after histological examination of the colon, when the pathologist suggested the possibility that this was metastatic carcinoma. The lesion shown in Figures 24.14 and 24.15 of a secondary mammary tumour in the femur was sent to the laboratory with no clinical details, and only on further enquiry, after histological examination of the section, did the history of a known primary mammary tumour emerge.

Metastases to the uterus from any primary site other than direct spread from adjacent pelvic organs is unusual. However, metastases can occur to the cervix, endometrium, and myometrium[12,13]. Secondary mammary carcinoma within the endometrium is illustrated in Figures 24.16 and 24.17. Another unusual site for metastatic tumour is within an existing tumour, for example a leiomyoma of the uterus[13]. A further example of this occurrence is shown in Figure 24.18, a typical meningioma in which sections showed the additional presence of metastatic mammary carcinoma. There have been several reports in the literature recently of endobronchial metastases from breast primaries[14,15]. On bronchoscopy these may resemble primary bronchial carcinoma, but a metastasis should always be considered in patients with a history of breast carcinoma who present with evidence of endobronchial disease.

Breast Cancer Presenting as an Axillary Lymph Node Metastasis

Between 0.5 and 1% of all patients with mammary carcinoma present with secondaries in an axillary lymph node. In some of these no breast lesion can be detected either by clinical or mammographic examination – although even then the most likely source of an axillary metastasis in a female is a primary tumour in the ipsilateral breast. The histological appearance of the metastatic lesion may strongly suggest primary origin within the breast and examples of typical metastases from both ductal and lobular carcinoma of the breast are illustrated in Chapter 19. However, the histological features are frequently less characteristic. Moreover other tumour types must also be considered. On the basis of histological examination and with the use of special stains, including immunohistochemical techniques and electron microscopy, it is usually possible to distinguish between metastatic tumour and lymphoma, to detect melanin in the case of a metastatic malignant melanoma, or to confirm the presence of mucin in metastatic adenocarcinoma[16]. Measurement of the oestrogen and progesterone receptors may also provide supporting evidence although, as mentioned previously, tumours other than primary breast carcinoma can contain hormone receptors.

If the lesion in the axillary lymph node proves to be a secondary carcinoma, and there is no clinically detectable primary in the breast, other sites of origin should be excluded. However, very extensive, detailed and exhaustive investigations are not justified because, by the time such a distant tumour has disseminated to produce a detectable axillary mass, the primary site will usually be apparent after a simple clinical search[17]. Moreover, prolonged investigations of other organs and systems may cause unnecessary delay in starting treatment. In the majority of patients in whom no other primary neoplasm is obvious, a carcinoma can be found in the mastectomy specimen. These small occult tumours are usually in the upper outer quadrant, and are sometimes found in the axillary tail. Occasionally, only *in situ* carcinoma can be demonstrated[18]. In the small percentage of cases in which no primary tumour is found in the breast it is possible that the primary site is indeed elsewhere. It is more likely, however, that the lesion is either so small that it was not detected on pathological examination, or that the original biopsy from the axilla represented a primary tumour in the axillary tail and not a metastasis. Other more remote possibilities are that carcinoma could arise in a benign epithelial inclusion in the lymph node, or that a primary tumour of the breast could regress. Patients who present with an axillary node metastasis and an occult breast carcinoma do no worse than other patients with positive axillary nodes, and indeed in several reported series their survival is better than the majority of patients with axillary node metastases[19,20].

References

1. McIntosh, I. H., Hooper, A. A., Millis, R. R. and Greening, W. P. (1976). Metastatic carcinoma within the breast. *Clin. Oncol.*, **2**, 393–401
2. Sandison, A. T. (1959). Metastatic tumours in the breast. *Br. J. Surg.*, **47**, 54–58
3. Nielsen, M., Andersen, J. A., Henriksen, F. W., Kristensen, P. B., Lorentzen, M., Ravn, V., Schiodt, T., Thorborg, J. V. and Ornvold, K. (1981). Metastases to the breast from extra-mammary carcinomas. *Acta Pathol. Microbiol. Scand. (Sect. A.)*, **89**, 251–256
4. Paulus, D. D. and Libshitz, H. I., (1982). Metastasis to the breast. *Radiol. Clin. N. Am.*, **20**, 561–568
5. Kashlan, R. B., Powell, R. W. and Nolting, S. F. (1982). Carcinoid and other tumors metastatic to the breast. *J. Surg. Oncol.*, **20**, 25–30
6. Lowden, R. G. and Taylor, H. B. (1974). Angioblastic meningioma with metastasis to the breast. *Arch. Pathol.*, **98**, 373–375
7. Azzopardi, J. G. and Eusebi, V. (1977). Melanocyte colonization and pigmentation of breast carcinoma. *Histopathology*, **1**, 21–30
8. Choudhury, M., DeRosas, J., Papsidero, L., Wajsman, Z., Beckley, S. and Pontes, J. E. (1982). Metastatic prostatic carcinoma to breast or primary breast carcinoma? *Urology*, **19**, 297–299
9. Salyer, W. R. and Salyer, D. C. (1973). Metastases of prostatic carcinoma to the breast. *J. Urol.*, **109**, 671–675
10. Chang, S. F., Burrell, M. I., Brand, M. H. and Garsten, J. J. (1978). The protean gastrointestinal manifestations of metastatic breast carcinoma. *Radiology*, **126**, 611–617
11. Rees, B. I. Okwonga, W. and Jenkins, I. L. (1976). Intestinal metastases from carcinoma of the breast. *Clin. Oncol.*, **2**, 113–119
12. Alcena, V. and Greenwald, E. S. (1977). Metastatic breast cancer. Pelvic and abdominal complications. *NY State J. Med.*, **77**, 1768–1773
13. Kumar, N. B. and Hart, W. R. (1982). Metastases to the uterine corpus from extragenital cancers: a clinicopathologic study of 63 cases. *Cancer*, **50**, 2163–2169
14. McNamee, M. J. and Scherzer, H. H. (1982). Endobronchial involvement in metastatic breast carcinoma. *Connecticut Med.*, **46**, 244–248

15. Albertini, R.E. and Ekberg, N.L. (1980). Endobronchial metastasis in breast cancer. *Thorax,* **35**, 435–440

16. Iglehart, J.D., Ferguson, B.J., Shingleton, W.W., Sabiston, D.C. Jr., Silva, J.S., Fetter, B.F. and McCarty, K.S. Jr. (1982). An ultrastructural analysis of breast carcinoma presenting as isolated axillary adenopathy. *Ann. Surg.,* **196**, 8–13

17. Patel, J., Nemoto, T., Rosner, D., Dao, T.L. and Pickren, J.W. (1981). Axillary lymph node metastasis from an occult breast cancer. *Cancer,* **47**, 2923–2927

18. Rosen, P.P. (1980). Axillary lymph node metastases in patients with occult noninvasive breast carcinoma. *Cancer,* **46**, 1298–1306

19. Ashikari, R., Rosen, P.P., Urban, J.A. and Senoo, T. (1976). Breast cancer presenting as an axillary mass. *Ann. Surg.,* **183**, 415–417

20. Vezzoni, P., Balestrazzi, A., Bignami, P., Concolino, F., Gennari, L. and Veronesi, U. (1979). Axillary lymph node metastases from occult carcinoma of the breast. *Tumori,* **65**, 87–91

Figures 24.13–24.18 will be found overleaf.

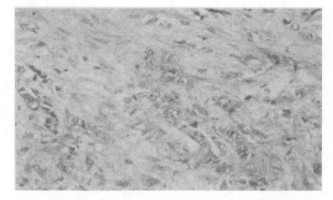

Figure 24.13 Lobular carcinoma of breast, metastatic to colon. From the same lesion as illustrated in Figures 24.11 and 24.12. The tumour cells contain red-staining intracytoplasmic mucin droplets. PAS after diastase digestion × 240

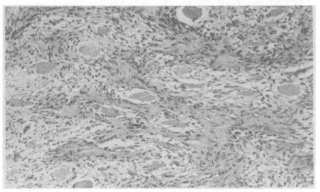

Figure 24.14 Mammary carcinoma, metastatic to femur. Section from the site of a pathological facture of the femur. The patient was known to have carcinoma of the breast. Much of the lesion comprised highly-cellular callus, and multiple sections were studied before secondary carcinoma was identified. The photograph shows reparative osteogenic tissue which has extended beyond the ruptured periosteum and is proliferating amongst the striated muscle of the thigh. H & E × 96

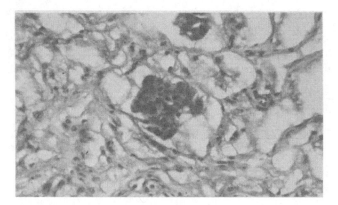

Figure 24.15 Mammary carcinoma, metastatic to femur. A further section from the lesion illustrated in Figure 24.14. This shows clusters of carcinoma cells with both intracellular and extracellular mucin, stained red. PAS after diastase digestion × 240

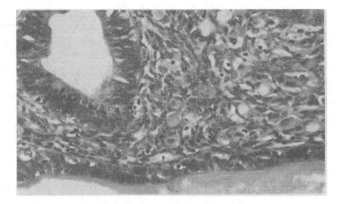

Figure 24.16 Endometrium: metastatic lobular carcinoma of the breast. Section of endometrial curettings from a patient with known lobular carcinoma of the breast. Intermingled with the spindle shaped cells of the stroma, there are spheroidal cells, some with eosinophilic cytoplasm, and others vacuolated and of 'signet-ring' appearance. H & E × 240

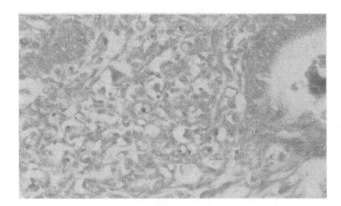

Figure 24.17 Endometrium: metastatic lobular carcinoma of the breast. A further section of the lesion illustrated in Figure 24.16, stained with Alcian blue to show the intracytoplasmic mucin of the carcinoma cells. Alcian blue/Neutral red × 240

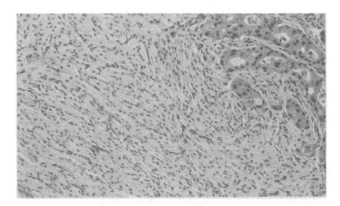

Figure 24.18 Mammary carcinoma, metastatic to an intracranial meningioma. From a patient who developed a space-occupying lesion of the brain, 2 years after mammary carcinoma had been diagnosed. Macroscopically, the intracranial lesion was a typical meningioma. The section shows secondary carcinoma, with tubular differentiation, in the top right-hand corner. The rest of the field is occupied by meningiomatous tissue. H & E × 96

Index